COLOR ATLAS
SYNOPSIS
CLINICAL
OPHTHALMOLOGY

WILLS EYE HOSPITAL

CORNEA

COLOR ATLAS AND SYNOPSIS OF CLINICAL OPHTHALMOLOGY SERIES

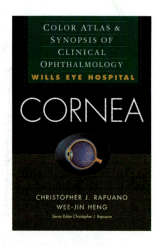

CORNEA
Christopher J. Rapuano, MD
Wee-Jin Heng, MD
0-07-137589-9

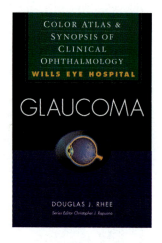

GLAUCOMA
Douglas J. Rhee, MD
0-07-137597-X

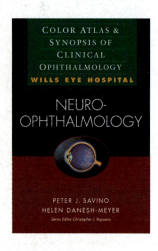

NEUROOPHTHALMOLOGY
Peter J. Savino, MD
Helen Danesh-Meyer, MD
0-07-137595-3

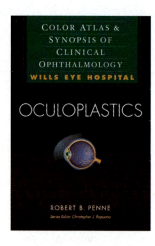

OCULOPLASTICS
Robert B. Penne, MD
0-07-137594-5

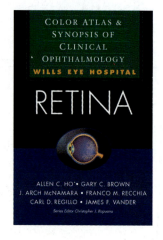

RETINA
Allen C. Ho, MD
Gary C. Brown, MD
J. Arch McNamara, MD
Franco M. Recchia, MD
Carl D. Regillo, MD
James F. Vander, MD
0-07-137596-1

COLOR ATLAS & SYNOPSIS OF CLINICAL OPHTHALMOLOGY

WILLS EYE HOSPITAL

CORNEA

Christopher J. Rapuano, MD
Professor of Ophthalmology
Jefferson Medical College of Thomas Jefferson University
Cornea Service
Wills Eye Hospital
Philadelphia, Pennsylvania

Wee-Jin Heng, MD
Associate Consultant
Department of Ophthalmology
Tan Tock Seng Hospital
Singapore

McGraw-Hill
MEDICAL PUBLISHING DIVISION

New York   Chicago   San Francisco   Lisbon   London   Madrid   Mexico City
Milan   New Delhi   San Juan   Seoul   Singapore   Sydney   Toronto

*The **McGraw·Hill** Companies*

Cornea: Color Atlas and Synopsis of Clinical Ophthalmology

Copyright © 2003 by The **McGraw-Hill** Companies, Inc. All rights reserved. Printed in Singapore. Except as permitted under the United States Copyright Act of 1976, no part of this publication may be reproduced or distributed in any form or by any means, or stored in a data base or retrieval system, without the prior written permission of the publisher.

1234567890   IMA/IMA   098765432

ISBN 0-07-137589-9

This book was set in Times Roman by Circle Graphics.
The editors were Darlene Barela Cooke, Susan J. Noujaim, and Karen Davis.
The production supervisor was Philip Galea.
The cover designer was Mary Belibasakis.
The index was prepared by Maria Coughlin, Editorial Services.
The printer and binder was Imago (U.S.A.), Inc., in Singapore.

This book is printed on acid-free paper.

Library of Congress Cataloging-in-Publication Data

Rapuano, Christopher J.
     Cornea : Color atlas and synopsis of clinical ophthalmology / Christopher J. Rapuano, Wee-Jin Heng.
         p.; cm.—(Color atlas and synopsis of clinical ophthalmology series)
     Includes bibliographical references and index.
     ISBN 0-07-137589-9
     1. Cornea—Diseases—Atlases. 2. Cornea—Diseases—Handbooks, manuals, etc. I. Heng, Wee-Jin. II. Title. III. Series.
     [DNLM: 1. Corneal Diseases—Atlases. WW 17 R221c 2003]
RE336 .R37   2003
617.7′19—dc21   2002075396

To my wonderful wife
Sara
an essential partner at home and at work; we make a perfect team

our children
Michael, Patrick, Daniel, and Megan
for continuing to remind me what is important in life

my parents
Cathie and Al
for all their love and support over the years

my three brothers, sisters-in-law, brother-in-law and their children, who demonstrate how essential family really is in our lives

Christopher J. Rapuano

To my beloved wife,
Elisa

our adorable children,
Jia-Hui, Jia-Ming, and Jia-Yuan

my dear parents,
Ann-Naa and Koon-Gek
for their unfailing love, understanding, and support

Wee-Jin Heng

TABLE OF CONTENTS

ABOUT THE SERIES

The beauty of the atlas/synopsis concept is the powerful combination of illustrative photographs and a summary approach to the text. Ophthalmology is a very visual discipline which lends itself nicely to clinical photographs. While the five ophthalmic subspecialties in this series, Cornea, Retina, Glaucoma, Oculoplastics, and Neuroophthalmology, employ varying levels of visual recognition, a relatively standard format for the text is used for all volumes.

The goal of the series is to provide an up-to-date clinical overview of the major areas of ophthalmology for students, residents, and practitioners in all the healthcare professions. The abundance of large, excellent quality photographs and concise, outline-form text will help achieve that objective.

Christopher J. Rapuano, MD
Series Editor

PREFACE

The main objective of basic ophthalmic education is to train the user to discover the full history of the patient's illness, recognize the abnormal physical signs, make a diagnosis, and suggest appropriate methods of treatment. The aim of higher training is to amplify these capabilities in breadth and depth through practical experience and subspecialty training. During case presentations and even clinical examinations, it is not uncommon to encounter residents making the wrong diagnosis and arriving at the wrong treatment plan. There are two principal reasons for this error. First, they may fail to detect all the abnormal signs and, second, they are unable to integrate and interpret the facts that are collected. The first step in the management of any condition is making a correct diagnosis. One must be able to detect all the abnormal signs and know what one is observing.

Our goal is to use color photographs of the important corneal, anterior segment, and external diseases with outline-form text to succinctly illustrate and describe these conditions. This atlas is intended not only for ophthalmic residents and cornea fellows but also for practicing physicians. Each section covers the clinical features of the important cornea and external eye diseases, diagnostic tests, differential diagnoses, and treatment. In addition to providing practical information on the approach and management of each condition, this book aids recognition of clinical signs by including a selection of classical photographs. In the field of cornea study, the old saying "a picture is worth a thousand words" does not apply since not even a thousand words can substitute for a good picture of the condition. The extensive use of color photographs throughout this affordable atlas will hopefully have a great impact on the memory and facilitate learning.

To emphasize the importance of sign recognition and the powers of observation, the following quotations may serve as useful reminders for all of us:

> Credit must be given to observation rather than theories, and to theories only in so far as they are confirmed by the observed facts.
> *Aristotle*

> The more I see, the more I see there is to see.
> *John Sebastian*

CHRISTOPHER J. RAPUANO, MD
WEE-JIN HENG, MD

ACKNOWLEDGMENTS

We would like to acknowledge the many people who helped make this book a reality. Most of the clinical photographs came from our patients. We are grateful to them for allowing us to subject them to flash photography. Several colleagues generously supplied additional photos including my partners Elisabeth Cohen, MD, and Peter Laibson, MD, two other Wills Eye Hospital Cornea Service members, Irving Raber, MD, and Sadeer Hannush, MD, and also Rolande Michaud, MD, via Patricia Laughrea, MD, from Quebec, Canada. We are, as always, eternally grateful to Elisabeth Cohen, the Chief of the Cornea Service at Wills Eye Hospital, for her constant support and great help in reviewing the text.

We also thank Bob Curtin, Jack Scully, and Roger Barone of the Audio-Visual Department at Wills Eye Hospital for all their help and expertise with the photographic needs for this book and all the books in this series.

We wish to thank Darlene Cooke, Kitty McCullough, and the team at McGraw-Hill for giving us the opportunity to be part of this series and for keeping the process moving forward.

We also wish to thank all of our fellows and residents, past and present, for all they do to encourage us to continue teaching and learning in our wonderful subspecialty of cornea and anterior segment disease.

COLOR ATLAS & SYNOPSIS OF CLINICAL OPHTHALMOLOGY

WILLS EYE HOSPITAL

CORNEA

Chapter 1

CONJUNCTIVAL INFECTIONS AND INFLAMMATIONS

BLEPHARITIS/MEIBOMITIS

Chronic blepharitis and meibomitis are very common, bilateral inflammations of the eyelid margins that may cause nonspecific ocular irritation which is often worse in the morning. On the other hand, some patients have severe blepharitis but no symptoms.

Etiology

- Staphylococcal infection, acne rosacea, seborrheic dermatitis

Symptoms

- Burning, itching, discomfort, foreign body sensation, tearing, crusting, mild discharge

Signs

- Associated atopic and seborrheic dermatitis, and ocular rosacea
- Hyperemia, telangiectasia, crusting, scaling, formation of collarettes around bases of lashes (staphylococcal), sleeves along eyelashes (seborrheic), and pouting of meibomian gland orifices, which can be expressed to produce a thickened lipid secretion, sometimes of toothpaste-like consistency (Figures 1-1A,B)
- Frothy and foamy tear film, conjunctival injection, inferior superficial punctate keratopathy, phlyctenulosis, corneal infiltrates

Treatment

- Warm compresses 10 minutes bid, eyelid margin scrubs with mild detergents
- Tear supplements while awake, topical erythromycin, bacitracin, or tetracycline ointment at bedtime
- Oral tetracycline 250 mg qid or doxycycline 100 mg bid in severe or recurrent cases. These medications can often be tapered to a much lower dose for long-term use (e.g., doxycycline 20 mg bid). Oral erythromycin (approximately 200 mg/d) can be used for children
- Judicious short-term use of topical corticosteroids for phlyctenulosis or infiltrates

Prognosis

- Good for significant improvement in symptoms over weeks, but the conditions are controlled rather than cured

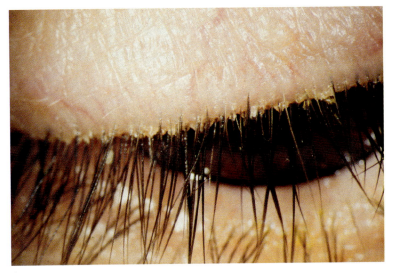

A

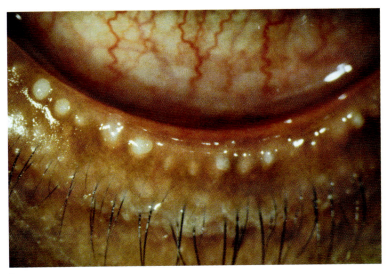

B

Figure 1-1 **Blepharitis** **A.** *Significant crusting at the base of the eyelashes is seen. A few collarettes are present.* **Meibomitis** **B.** *Severe pouting of the meibomian glands of the inferior eyelid can be seen. The eyelid margin is thickened and inflamed, with some conjunctival injection visible.*

CHALAZION (INTERNAL HORDEOLUM, STYE)

A chalazion is tender eyelid mass, often with surrounding erythema and swelling. It may be small or large, and when severe can cause significant eyelid inflammation.

Etiology

- Blockage of meibomian gland orifices and stagnation of sebaceous secretions
- Associated with blepharitis/meibomitis and acne rosacea

Symptoms

- Eyelid swelling, pain, and redness. Often a history of previous chalazia. Rarely, large, central chalazia can cause corneal flattening, especially after refractive surgery or induced astigmatism

Signs

- Subcutaneous round, firm, swelling in the tarsal plate. May have an associated pyogenic granuloma on eversion of eyelid (Figures 1-2A,B)
- Sometimes may be associated with significant eyelid inflammation (preseptal cellulitis)

Differential Diagnosis

- External hordeolum: an acute staphylococcal infection of a lash follicle and its associated gland of Zeis or Moll
- Pyogenic granuloma: a vascularized mass protruding from the conjunctiva
- Sebaceous gland carcinoma: suspect in recurrent chalazia, eyelid margin excoriation, or loss of lashes, especially if unilateral

Diagnosis

- Eyelid biopsy if suspicious of sebaceous gland carcinoma

Treatment

- Warm compresses, eyelid massage and hygiene
- Topical erythromycin, bacitracin, or tetracycline ointment for blepharitis/meibomitis
- Oral tetracycline 250 mg qid or doxycycline 100 mg bid in inflamed, severe, or recurrent cases, to prevent recurrent chalazia
- Corticosteroid injection can be considered to reduce scarring in recalcitrant cases
- Incision and curettage if no improvement with medical treatment

Prognosis

- Very good with medical treatment. If unsuccessful, surgical treatment is quite effective.

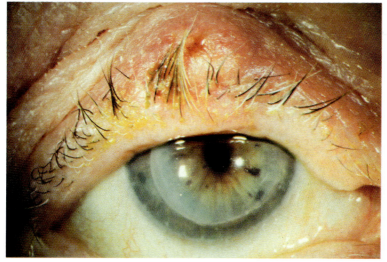

A

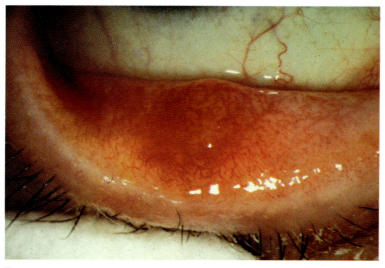

B

Figure 1-2 Chalazion **A.** *A large, inflamed chalazion of the upper eyelid. Severe blepharitis and crusting of the eyelid margin, predisposing factors for development of chalazia, are also present.* **B.** *Lower eyelid eversion reveals a large indurated mass consistent with a chalazion.*

BACTERIAL CONJUNCTIVITIS (NONGONOCOCCAL)

Bacterial conjunctivitis is a relatively uncommon, usually bilateral condition, characterized by a mucopurulent or purulent discharge.

Etiology

- *Staphylococcus aureus, Staphylococcus epidermidis*
- *Streptococcus pneumoniae*
- *Haemophilus influenzae* (especially in children), others

Symptoms

- Redness, discharge, foreign body sensation, burning, itchiness, photophobia

Signs

- Purulent or mucopurulent discharge (Figure 1-3)
- Conjunctival hyperemia, maximal in the fornices
- Pseudomembranes may be present in severe infections
- Punctate epitheliopathy
- Preauricular lymphadenopathy is usually absent

Diagnosis

- Conjunctival swab for Gram's stain, cultures, and sensitivities if severe

Treatment

- Spontaneous resolution in days to 1 to 2 weeks is usual
- Tear supplement to wash away discharge
- Empiric broad-spectrum topical antibiotic drops (e.g., polymyxin/trimethoprim [e.g. Polytrim®], fluoroquinolones, gentamicin, tobramycin, neomycin/gramicidin/bacitracin [e.g., Neosporin®]) qid for 1 week
- Antibiotic ointments (e.g., fluoroquinolones, tobramycin, tetracycline, bacitracin, neomycin/polymyxin/bacitracin [e.g., Neosporin®]) can be used qid for 1 week in patients in whom the drops wash out very quickly, such as crying children

Prognosis

- Very good. Severe infections can cause permanent conjunctival scarring.

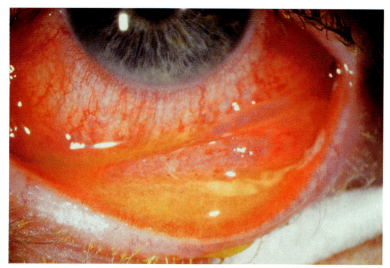

Figure 1-3 Bacterial conjunctivitis *Diffuse conjunctival injection and a purulent discharge is present in this eye with bacterial conjunctivitis.*

GONOCOCCAL BACTERIAL CONJUNCTIVITIS

Gonococcal conjunctivitis is a rare, occasionally bilateral condition, characterized by acute onset of a severe purulent discharge.

Etiology

- Primarily *Neisseria gonorrhoeae*
- Occasionally *Neisseria meningitidis*
- It is typically sexually transmitted

Symptoms

- Redness, severe purulent discharge, foreign body sensation, burning, photophobia

Signs

- Severe purulent discharge with a hyperacute onset (within 12 to 24 h); pseudomembranes may be present
- Marked conjunctival inflammation and chemosis (Figure 1-4)
- Eyelid swelling
- Preauricular lymphadenopathy is often present
- Punctate epitheliopathy, corneal epithelial defect, infiltrate, ulcer, or perforation

Diagnosis

- Conjunctival scraping for immediate Gram's stain, cultures, and sensitivities. The diagnosis is confirmed if the Gram stain demonstrates gram-negative intracellular diplococci.

Treatment

- Systemic ceftriaxone 1 g IM in a single dose if there is no corneal involvement. If the patient is allergic to cephalosporins, fluoroquinolones are the drugs of choice.
- If there is corneal involvement or corneal involvement cannot be excluded due to a limited slit-lamp examination, the patient should be treated with ceftriaxone 1 g IV q 12 to 24 h for 3 days.
- Topical ciprofloxacin drops q 2 h, or q 1 h if the cornea is involved.
- Ocular irrigation with saline qid to q 2 h to eliminate the discharge.
- Evaluate and treat for possible coinfection with *Chlamydia* (e.g., azithromycin 1 g po once).
- Evaluate sexual partners for sexually transmitted diseases.

Prognosis

- Very good if diagnosed and treated appropriately before corneal involvement occurs. If the cornea is involved, the prognosis is guarded.

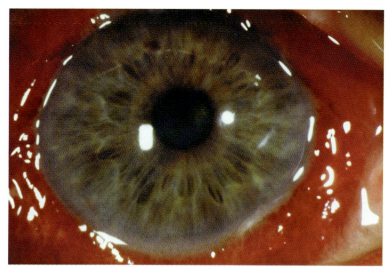

Figure 1-4 Gonococcal conjunctivitis *Severe inflammation and chemosis is present throughout the conjunctiva in this right eye. Some purulent discharge is present on the eyelid and conjunctiva nasally. The cornea is not involved.*

VIRAL CONJUNCTIVITIS (TYPICALLY ADENOVIRUS)

Viral conjunctivitis is a common, very contagious, usually bilateral condition, characterized by the rapid onset of redness, itchiness, and tearing, first in one eye and then the other.

Etiology

Adenovirus Serotypes 8, 19   Epidemic keratoconjunctivitis

Adenovirus Serotypes 3, 7   Pharyngoconjunctival fever, usually in children

Others   Herpes simplex virus, enteroviruses, Newcastle disease virus, Epstein-Barr virus

Symptoms

- Tearing, itching, burning, redness, foreign body sensation, photophobia
- History of contact with someone with a red eye, recent upper respiratory tract infection, or recent eye examination

Signs

- Eyelid edema
- Watery discharge
- Generalized conjunctival hyperemia, subconjunctival hemorrhages
- Conjunctival follicles, which are frequently most apparent in the inferior fornices (Figure 1-5A)
- Membranes or pseudomembranes in severe cases
- Conjunctival membranes consist of coagulated exudate adherent to inflamed conjunctival epithelium. Clinically, a true membrane causes bleeding upon attempted removal and a pseudomembrane does not, but this rule is not universal. The causes of true membranes and pseudomembranes are similar
- Central punctate epithelial keratitis, and occasionally an epithelial defect (Figure 1-5B)
- Preauricular lymphadenopathy is often present.
- Subepithelial infiltrates (SEIs) can occur days to weeks after the onset of the acute infection (Figure 1-5C)

Treatment

- Artificial tears and cool compresses 4 to 8 times a day.
- Antihistamines (e.g., antazoline, naphazoline) qid for itching.
- Removal of membranes or pseudomembranes.
- Corticosteroid drops in severe cases with membranes or pseudomembranes or erosions. A long, slow taper of mild corticosteroid drops can be used in eyes with SEIs that affect visual function.
- Strict observation of hygienic measures is needed to avoid spreading the infection.

Prognosis

- Very good. If clinically significant subepithelial infiltrates develop, the treatment course can be prolonged. Severe infections with membranes or pseudomembranes can cause permanent conjunctival scarring.

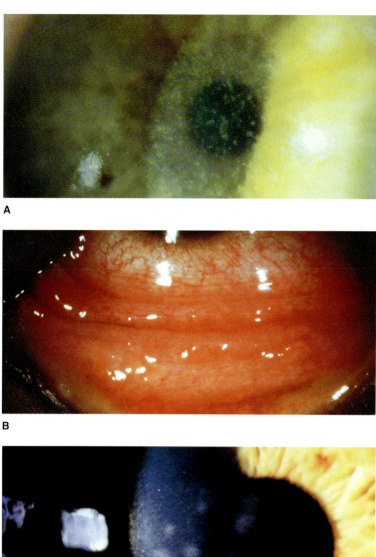

Figure 1-5   Viral conjunctivitis   A. *A central punctate epithelial keratitis as seen in this eye is often found early in the course of viral conjunctivitis, most commonly caused by adenovirus.* **B.** *Diffuse conjunctival injection with a severe follicular reaction, greatest inferiorly, is present in this eye with viral conjunctivitis.* **C.** *Multiple subepithelial infiltrates (SEIs) of the cornea can be seen 2 months after resolution of adenoviral keratoconjunctivitis. These SEIs tend to resolve on their own. If severe, they can affect visual acuity and cause glare symptoms. SEIs generally respond to low-dose topical steroid drops; however, if started, these drops need to be tapered very slowly, over months.*

CHLAMYDIAL CONJUNCTIVITIS (ADULT INCLUSION CONJUNCTIVITIS)

Adult chlamydial conjunctivitis is a relatively common, usually unilateral condition that is transmitted sexually and typically affects young adults.

Etiology

- *Chlamydia trachomatis* serotypes D through K
- Typically sexually transmitted

Symptoms

- Tearing, itching, burning, redness, foreign body sensation, photophobia, discharge of longer than 3 to 4 weeks' duration
- May be associated with urethritis, vaginitis, or cervicitis

Signs

- Stringy, white mucopurulent discharge
- Large follicles in the inferior fornices (Figure 1-6)
- Superior tarsal follicles, occasionally follicles at the limbus
- Superior limbal or peripheral nummular corneal infiltrates and pannus
- Mild preauricular lymphadenopathy may be present

Diagnosis

- History of sexual exposure, concomitant genitourinary symptoms
- Direct immunofluorescent antibody test of conjunctival smears
- Giemsa stain cytology for basophilic cytoplasmic inclusion bodies of Halberstedter-Prowazek; more common in newborns than adults
- McCoy chlamydial cell culture

Treatment

- Azithromycin 1 g po once, doxycycline 100 mg po bid, or tetracycline, erythromycin or clarithromycin 250 mg qid for 2 to 6 weeks.
- Topical tetracycline or erythromycin ointment qid for 4 to 6 weeks.
- Referral for treatment of sexual partners and other sexually transmitted diseases should be done.

Prognosis

- Very good

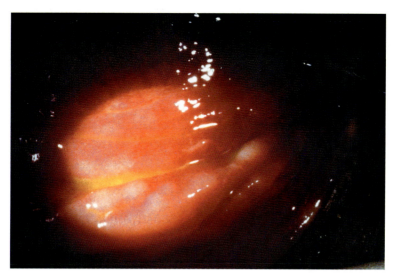

Figure 1-6   Chlamydial conjunctivitis   *A severe inferior conjunctival follicular reaction can be seen in this eye with chronic chlamydial conjunctivitis. There were similar conjunctival follicles superiorly. There is also diffuse bulbar conjunctival injection.*

TRACHOMA

Trachoma is a bilateral conjunctivitis that is common in underdeveloped countries where hygiene is poor. It is endemic in Africa and certain parts of Asia and is the most common cause of preventable blindness, affecting millions of people around the world.

Etiology

- *Chlamydia trachomatis* serotypes A, B, Ba, and C

Signs

World Health Organization Classification

- *TF* (trachomatous follicular inflammation): more than 5 follicles greater than 0.5 mm on the upper tarsus
- *TI* (trachomatous intense inflammation): thickening obscuring more than 50% of tarsal vessels
- *TS* (trachomatous scarring): cicatrization with white lines or bands in tarsal conjunctiva (Arlt's line) (Figure 1-7)
- *TT* (trachomatous trichiasis): trichiasis of at least 1 eyelash
- *CO* (corneal opacity): corneal opacity involving at least part of the pupillary margin
- Cicatrization of limbal follicles results in depressions known as Herbert's pits.

Diagnosis

- Diagnostic investigation is similar to that for adult inclusion conjunctivitis.

Treatment

- SAFE strategy: *s*urgery for trichiasis, *a*ntibiotics (repeated every 6 to 12 months in endemic areas), *f*acial and *e*nvironmental hygiene
- Antibiotic treatment similar to that for adult inclusion conjunctivitis

Prognosis

- Very good unless significant corneal scarring has developed. Reinfection is common if hygienic conditions do not improve.

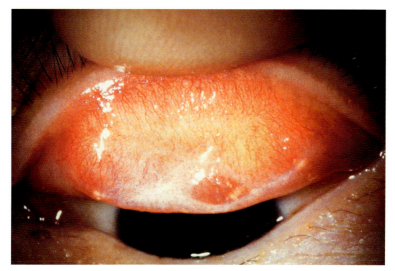

Figure 1-7   Trachoma   *White scarring of the superior tarsal conjunctiva is present. The white line is called an Arlt's line.*

MOLLUSCUM CONTAGIOSUM

Molluscum contagiosum is an uncommon cause of chronic follicular conjunctivitis, which is usually unilateral and may be missed if the eyelid margin is not examined closely.

Etiology

- Viral particles from molluscum contagiosum lesions of the eyelid may cause a toxic response of the conjunctiva.

Symptoms

- Tearing, itching, burning, redness, foreign body sensation. May be chronic.

Signs

- Single or multiple, dome-shaped, umbilicated, molluscum contagiosum eyelid lesions associated with follicular conjunctivitis. May be chronic (Figures 1-8A,B).
- Watery or mucoid discharge

- Corneal micropannus if longstanding
- In immunocompromised patients, there may be extensive eyelid lesions with minimal conjunctival inflammation.

Treatment

- Removal of eyelid lesion by shaving excision, incision and curettage, cauterization, or cryotherapy
- If severe, consider a work-up for an immune deficiency disorder such as HIV infection.

Prognosis

- Very good, but it can take many weeks for the follicular conjunctivitis to resolve after the lesion is treated.

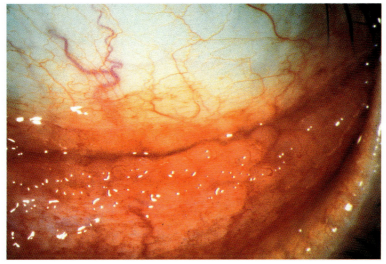

A

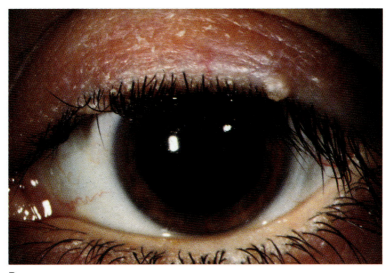

B

Figure 1-8   Molluscum contagiosum   A. *A severe inferior palpebral conjunctival follicular reaction of several months duration is apparent. Generally the bulbar conjunctiva is much less injected.* **B.** *In the patient seen in Figure 1-8A, an umbilicated creamy colored nodule is seen at the upper eyelid margin. If not searched for carefully, molluscum contagiosum lesions can easily be overlooked. Small incision and curettage into the center of the lesion, causing bleeding, is often curative.*

LIGNEOUS CONJUNCTIVITIS

Ligneous disease is a very rare cause of chronic unilateral or bilateral conjunctivitis with characteristic "woody," thick membrane formation.

Etiology

- Likely due to an inherited plasminogen deficiency

Symptoms

- Tearing, itching, burning, redness, foreign body sensation. May note an eyelid mass. Generally chronic.

Signs

- Chronic conjunctivitis with wood-like, thick membrane formation on the upper tarsus and occasionally the lower tarsus (Figure 1-9)
- May have similar involvement of the mouth, nasopharynx, trachea, and genitourinary mucous membranes.

Treatment

- Removal of pseudomembranes
- Topical cyclosporine, hyaluronidase, or corticosteroids
- Topical or systemic lys-plasminogen replacement therapy may be beneficial

Prognosis

- Poor with previous treatments. Topical or systemic lys-plasminogen replacement therapy is a promising new development for this rare condition.

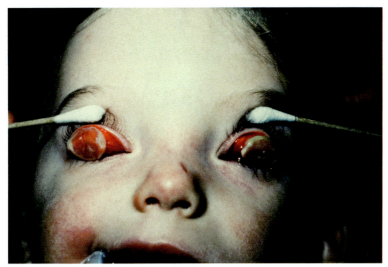

Figure 1-9 Ligneous conjunctivitis *Prominent white, "woody" membranes attached to the superior palpebral conjunctivas of both eyes are present in this baby with ligneous conjunctivitis. (Photo courtesy of Rolande Michaud, MD.)*

PEDICULOSIS

Pediculosis is a sexually transmitted disease caused by contact with pubic lice.

Etiology

- Eyelid infection with pubic lice. May be unilateral or bilateral.

Symptoms

- Tearing, itching, burning, redness, foreign body sensation. May be chronic.

Signs

- Lice, nits (eggs), and blood-tinged debris on eyelids and lashes (Figure 1-10)
- Mild to severe chronic follicular conjunctivitis

Treatment

- Remove all lice and nits under slit-lamp illumination.
- Topical antibiotic ointment (e.g., tetracycline, bacitracin, or erythromycin) on eyelids tid for 1 to 2 weeks to smother the lice and nits.
- Oral ivermectin, 2 doses, 1 week apart, has been shown to be effective.
- Antilice shampoo and lotion to treat nonocular areas. Wash and machine dry all clothes and linens.
- Treat sexual partners.

Prognosis

- Good if all the lice and nits are removed. Reinfection can occur if sexual partners and clothes and linens are not treated appropriately.

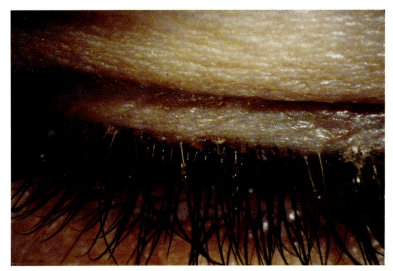

Figure 1-10 Pediculosis *Several lice can be seen attached to the base of the eyelashes in this left eye with pediculosis. The most obvious one is located temporally. Numerous tubular nits are present on the eyelash shafts. Some blood tinged debris can be seen at the base of the lashes.*

PARINAUD'S OCULOGLANDULAR SYNDROME

Parinaud's oculoglandular syndrome is an uncommon, usually unilateral condition with diverse causes, characterized by conjunctival granulomas and extremely swollen preauricular and submandibular lymph nodes.

Etiology

- Cat-scratch fever is the most common cause.
- Mononucleosis
- Tularemia
- Tuberculosis
- Rare causes: sporotrichosis, syphilis, coccidioidomycosis, chancroid, lymphogranuloma venereum

Symptoms

- Redness, foreign body sensation, discharge
- Fever, malaise, skin rash

Signs

- Unilateral conjunctival granulomas and large follicles (Figure 1-11)
- Severe ipsilateral preauricular or submandibular lymphadenopathy

Diagnosis

- Appropriate blood tests, conjunctival stains, cultures, and conjunctival biopsy
- Complete blood count, serology, and chest x-ray as needed

Treatment

- Topical antibiotic ointment (e.g., tetracycline, erythromycin, fluoroquinolone, bacitracin, polymyxin) for 4 weeks
- Systemic treatment varies according to cause.

Prognosis

- Generally good, although it depends on the specific etiology.

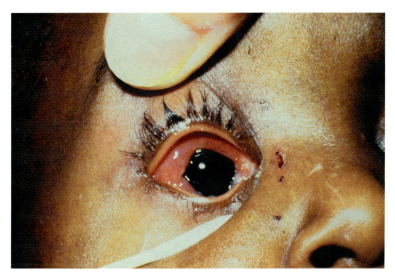

Figure 1-11   Parinaud's oculoglandular syndrome   *Severe diffuse conjunctival inflammation along with a superotemporal conjunctival granuloma is present in this child with cat scratch disease. Note the skin abrasions near the nose which were presumably caused by a cat scratch. (Photo courtesy of Peter Laibson, MD.)*

OPHTHALMIA NEONATORUM

Neonatal conjunctivitis (ophthalmia neonatorum) is unilateral or bilateral conjunctival inflammation occurring during the first month of life.

Etiology

Chemical Usually causes relatively mild diffuse injection without discharge which lasts no longer than 24 hours. Typically due to prophylactic silver nitrate drops.

Neisseria gonorrhoeae Causes copious purulent discharge which may be associated with membrane formation. Presents within first few days of life

Herpes Simplex Type 2 Associated with eyelid margin vesicles. Presents within 1 week of birth.

Chlamydia trachomatis Causes a purulent papillary conjunctivitis because the infant cannot produce follicles. May have pseudomembranes. Presents during the second week of life.

Simple Bacterial (e.g., *Staphylococcus, Streptococcus*, Gram-Negative Species) Presents within first few days after birth

Signs

- Eyelid edema, conjunctival injection, chemosis, purulent discharge (Figure 1-12)
- Keratitis is uncommon but may occur if treatment for gonococcal conjunctivitis is delayed.

Differential Diagnosis

- Nasolacrimal duct obstruction: tearing, nonpurulent discharge, and no infection.

Diagnosis

- Conjunctival scrapings for Gram's stain, Giemsa stain, bacterial culture, immunofluorescent tests, and viral culture
- Never assume only one pathogen is responsible.

Treatment

Empiric Topical tetracycline, ciprofloxacin, bacitracin, or erythromycin ointment qid and erythromycin 25 mg/kg po bid for 2 weeks

Chemical Artificial tears or no treatment

Neisseria gonorrhoeae Topical saline irrigation 4 to 8 times a day. Topical penicillin or ciprofloxacin q 1 h. Systemic single dose ceftriaxone 125 mg IM. Erythromycin 12.5 mg/ kg po qid for 2 weeks.

Herpes Simplex Type 2 Topical acyclovir (e.g., Zovirax®) or vidarabine (e.g., Vira-A®) ointment 5 times a day and taper over 1 week. Consider IV acyclovir.

Chlamydia trachomatis Topical tetracycline or erythromycin ointment qid and erythromycin 12.5 mg/kg po qid for 2 weeks.

Simple Bacterial Ciprofloxacin, bacitracin, gentamicin, or tobramycin ointment qid for 2 weeks

- Evaluate both parents for genital infection and treat accordingly.

Prognosis

- Generally good if diagnosed and treated appropriately before any corneal or systemic involvement occurs

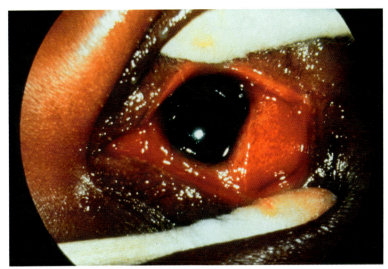

Figure 1-12   Ophthalmia neonatorum   *This infant had a severe diffuse conjunctivitis from a Chlamydia infection. (Photo courtesy of Irving Raber, MD.)*

ALLERGIC CONJUNCTIVITIS

Allergic conjunctivitis (e.g., hay fever conjunctivitis) is a very common type I hypersensitivity reaction causing conjunctival injection and itching that generally occurs during the hay fever season.

Etiology

- Pollen, grass, spores, hair, pets, wool, dust, etc.

Symptoms

- Itching, mucous discharge, tearing, redness, history of allergy. Symptoms are typically seasonal and vary with exposure.

Signs

- Eyelid edema
- Watery or mucoid discharge
- Conjunctival hyperemia with a mild papillary response
- Chemosis (Figure 1-13)
- The cornea is generally not involved.

Differential Diagnosis

- Perennial variant can occur at any time of the year.

Treatment

- Avoid exposure to offending allergen.
- Cool compresses, artificial tears
- Topical antihistamines (e.g., emedastine, levocabastine, naphazoline, antazoline) bid to qid
- Topical mast cell stabilizers (e.g., cromolyn, lodoxamide, olopatadine) bid to qid
- Oral antihistamine (e.g., diphenhydramine 25 mg po tid), especially if rhinitis is present
- Mild topical corticosteroid if severe (e.g., loteprednol 0.2%, fluorometholone 0.1%) qid for short duration
- Skin testing and desensitization therapy can be helpful in some cases.

Prognosis

- Good, but often mild chronic symptoms persist.

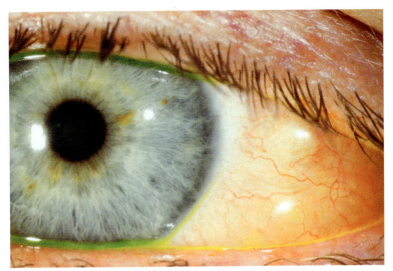

Figure 1-13 Allergic conjunctivitis *Conjunctival chemosis can be seen temporally due to an acute allergic reaction from cat fur touching the eye.*

ATOPIC KERATOCONJUNCTIVITIS

Atopic keratoconjunctivitis is an uncommon, bilateral perennial condition that may also involve the eyelids, and occurs primarily in patients with atopic dermatitis.

Etiology

- Chronic type I hypersensitivity allergic re-action similar to vernal keratoconjunctivitis, but causing more prominent eyelid and peri-orbital skin involvement

Symptoms

- Itching, tearing, redness, discharge
- History of atopy

Signs

- Eyelid crusting, eczema, and staphylococcal blepharitis (Figure 1-14)
- Mucoid discharge
- Small papillae on the palpebral conjunctiva with edema giving a velvety appearance
- Conjunctival scarring and symblepharon formation in advanced cases
- Corneal punctate epithelial erosions, vascularization
- May have associated keratoconus, cataract, and retinal detachment

Differential Diagnosis

- Differs from vernal keratoconjunctivitis in that atopic keratoconjunctivitis presents in adult life, papillae are small, there is an absence of limbitis and Trantas' dots, and it may cause neovascularization and cicatrization.

Treatment

- Cool compresses, artificial tears
- Topical mast cell stabilizers (e.g., cromolyn, lodoxamide, olopatadine) bid to qid
- Topical corticosteroid if severe (e.g., fluoro-metholone ointment bid on eyelids and/or loteprednol 0.2% to 0.5%, fluorometholone 0.1%, or prednisolone 0.125% to 1.0% drops qid) as short-term treatment
- An oral antihistamine may be helpful (e.g., diphenhydramine 25 mg po tid)
- Cyclosporine drops can have a corticosteroid-sparing effect in severe cases.

Prognosis

- Fair to good, depending on the severity of the condition. Must monitor intraocular pressure regularly, even if corticosteroids are used only on the eyelids.

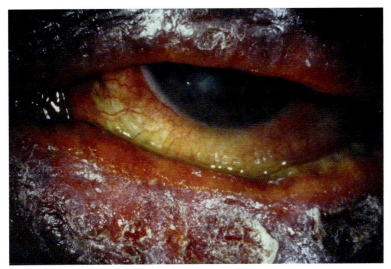

Figure 1-14   Atopic keratoconjunctivitis   *Eyelid erythema, thickening, and scaling are apparent in this patient with atopic disease. The skin has a leathery texture, and there is loss of lashes. Conjunctival injection and an old inferior corneal scar can be appreciated.*

VERNAL KERATOCONJUNCTIVITIS

Vernal keratoconjunctivitis (spring catarrh) is a seasonal, recurrent, bilateral, type I hypersensitivity reaction usually presenting in childhood and gradually resolving after puberty.

Etiology and Epidemiology

- Type I hypersensitivity allergic reaction similar to atopic keratoconjunctivitis, but with a seasonal exacerbation and less eyelid and skin involvement
- Males are affected more commonly than females.

Symptoms

- Itching, tearing, foreign body sensation, burning, discharge

Signs

- Stringy, mucopurulent discharge
- Milky-white pseudomembranes
- Superior tarsal papillae of medium to giant size, ptosis (Figure 1-15A)
- Occasionally, limbal papillae (limbitis) that may be associated with small white spots containing eosinophils (Trantas' dots) (Figure 1-15B).
- Superior corneal punctate epithelial erosions, corneal ulceration ("shield" ulcer)
- Mild subepithelial corneal scarring

Differential Diagnosis

- Giant papillary conjunctivitis (GPC) is much less severe, and is characterized by small- to medium-sized superior tarsal papillae. It can be unilateral or bilateral, depending on the cause. Also, GPC is caused by an allergic reaction to protein build-up on contact lenses, particularly soft lenses; ocular prosthetics; or protruding sutures following surgery.

Treatment

- If mild, treat as for atopic conjunctivitis.
- Mast cell stabilizers are effective, especially if initiated before the allergy season. They also have a corticosteroid-sparing function.
- If severe or in the presence of shield ulcer, use a short course of topical corticosteroids with antibiotic drops or ointments 4 to 6 times a day. Prolonged use of corticosteroid is discouraged and monitoring of intraocular pressure and lens clarity should be performed regularly.

Prognosis

- Fair to good, depending on the severity of the condition

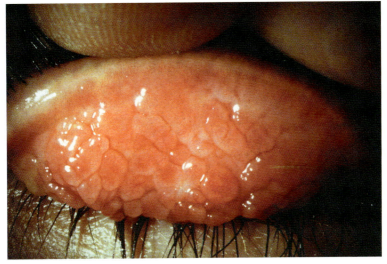

A

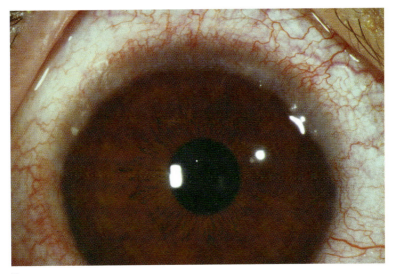

B

Figure 1-15   Vernal conjunctivitis   A. *Large, confluent papillae of the superior tarsal conjunctiva are present. These are flat-topped and are termed "cobblestone" papillae.* **B.** *Papillae can be more prominent at the limbus than the tarsal conjunctiva in certain patients, most commonly of African heritage. In these patients the condition is called "limbal vernal conjunctivitis" and the white spots are termed "Trantas' dots." In this patient, limbal follicles and Trantus' dots can be seen superiorly, especially at the 10 o'clock and 1 to 3 o'clock limbus.*

SUPERIOR LIMBIC KERATOCONJUNCTIVITIS

Superior limbic keratoconjunctivitis (SLK) is an uncommon, usually bilateral, relapsing, chronic inflammatory reaction that is frequently associated with thyroid dysfunction. It usually affects middle-aged females.

Etiology

- Unknown, but most likely related to mechanical trauma involving the superior palpebral and lax bulbar conjunctiva

Symptoms

- Foreign body sensation, burning, occasionally redness

Signs

- Hyperemia, thickening, redundance and laxity of superior bulbar conjunctiva (Figure 1-16A)
- Lack of luster and positive staining of superior bulbar conjunctiva with fluorescein and rose bengal dyes
- Fine, velvety, superior tarsal papillae
- Superior corneal filaments, punctate erosions, and occasionally pannus

Treatment

- Preservative-free artificial tear drops q 2 h. Consider temporary or permanent punctal occlusion.
- Acetylcysteine (e.g., Mucomyst®) 10% drops qid for treatment of corneal filaments. Topical mast cell stabilizers (e.g., cromolyn, lodoxamide, olopatadine bid to qid) can be helpful.
- Application of silver nitrate 0.5% *solution* to superior bulbar and palpebral conjunctiva for 15 seconds
- Local cautery or surgical resection of superior bulbar conjunctiva (Figure 1-16B)

Prognosis

- Good for improvement in symptoms, fair for complete resolution of symptoms. Can be recalcitrant to treatment.

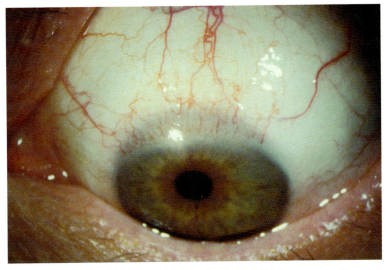

A

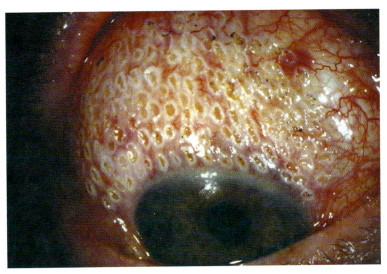

B

Figure 1-16 Superior limbic keratoconjunctivitis (SLK) A. *In SLK, there is localized conjunctival injection of the superior bulbar conjunctiva. There is pannus and thickened conjunctiva at the superior limbus.* **B.** *In the patient shown in Figure 1-16A, medical treatment failed. Localized conjunctival cautery after injection of local anesthesia was performed. This treatment is often successful in significantly improving the patient's symptoms.*

FLOPPY EYELID SYNDROME

Floppy eyelid syndrome, an uncommon condition, is due to a spontaneous eversion of the upper eyelid during sleep, thereby exposing the upper tarsal conjunctiva and cornea to trauma from pillows or bed linens. It typically affects obese men who have a history of sleep apnea.

Etiology

- An extremely lax, floppy upper eyelid everts, causing corneal exposure

Symptoms

- Chronic redness, foreign body sensation, discharge. Often worse in the morning.

Signs

- Easy eversion of upper eyelid. Tarsus feels soft and rubbery.
- Chronic papillary conjunctivitis of the upper tarsus, superficial punctate keratopathy (Figure 1-17)

Treatment

- Protect the eye by taping it closed or placing an eyeshield during sleep.
- Artificial tears or antibiotic ointment for lubrication, especially at bedtime
- A horizontal eyelid tightening procedure may be necessary to effect a permanent cure.

Prognosis

- Very good with a horizontal eyelid tightening procedure

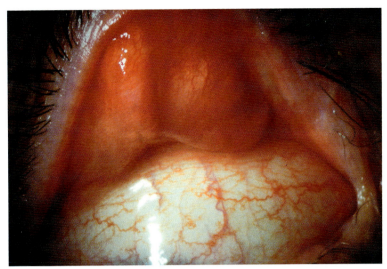

Figure 1-17   Floppy eyelid syndrome   *The superior eyelid is extremely lax and easily everted by pulling the eyelid margin superiorly. There is a fine, diffuse papillary reaction of the upper palpebral conjunctiva.*

TOXIC AND FACTITIOUS KERATOCONJUNCTIVITIS (KERATITIS MEDICAMENTOSA)

Chronic toxic conjunctivitis may be unilateral or bilateral, depending on the cause. Factitious conjunctivitis is caused by self-instillation of material to cause a reddened eye.

Etiology

- Aminoglycoside antibiotics, especially fortified medications
- Antiviral agents
- Glaucoma agents, particularly epinephrine, brimonidine, pilocarpine, carbonic anhydrase inhibitors
- Any preserved eyedrops
- Topical anesthetics
- Topical nonsteroidal anti-inflammatory agents
- Self-trauma, often for secondary gain, such as missing work or school

Differential Diagnosis

- Mucus fishing syndrome: a rare, unilateral or bilateral condition resulting from repeated self-traumatization of the conjunctiva while trying to remove mucus from the conjunctiva. Patients often do not admit to this activity unless pressed.

Symptoms

- Chronic redness, itching, foreign body sensation, mild discharge

Signs

- Initially a papillary conjunctival reaction, later followed by formation of follicles, predominantly involving the inferior fornices (Figure 1-18A)
- Inferior punctate epitheliopathy
- Inferior conjunctival erosions. Conjunctival necrosis can occur in severe cases.

- Severe corneal involvement may cause a sterile stromal ring infiltrate, that is sometimes mistaken for infectious keratitis, especially with anesthetic abuse (Figure 1-18B).
- Rarely, sterile corneal, conjunctival, or scleral melting can occur (Figure 1-18C).

Diagnosis

- Detailed history taking is most important.

Treatment

- Discontinue offending medication or self-abuse.
- Frequent preservative-free artificial tear drops 4 to 8 times a day
- Artificial tear or mild antibiotic ointment (e.g., erythromycin) if there is significant epitheliopathy
- Consider pressure patching (marking the patch to make sure it is not removed) for 1 to 2 days to prevent the patient from placing anything in the eye.
- Hospitalization may sometimes be required for patients unresponsive to treatment to ensure that they do not continue to use the offending medication or abuse the eye, especially for anesthetic abuse.

Prognosis

- Very good if the offending medication or self-abuse can be stopped before significant corneal damage has occurred.

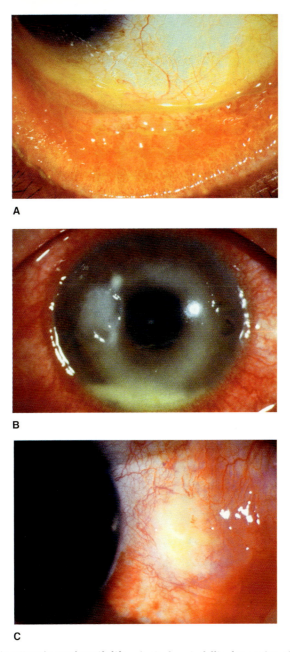

A

B

C

Figure 1-18   Toxic/allergic conjunctivitis   A. *A chronic follicular conjunctivitis secondary to an allergic reaction to topical apraclonidine (Iopidine®). It resolved over weeks once the medication was discontinued.* **Topical anesthetic abuse   B.** *This patient was treated for a fungal ulcer located from the 9 to 11 o'clock positions. It was resolving slowly until he stole proparacaine from the physician's office and developed a large ring infiltrate and hypopyon consistent with topical anesthetic abuse.* **Toxic/factitious keratoconjunctivitis   C.** *This eye has a localized conjunctival abrasion and injection. There is some associated subconjunctival hemorrhage. After obtaining a systemic work-up (which was negative), and trying several medical regimens without success, it was learned that the patient was poking herself in the eye with a needle to get out of work. She was referred for a psychological evaluation.*

OCULAR ROSACEA

Acne rosacea is a common skin disease of unknown etiology with frequent ocular involvement, typically occurring in middle-aged adults. It is often associated with dry eye syndrome.

Etiology

- Rosacea is an idiopathic dermatologic condition affecting the pilosebaceous units of the facial and eyelid skin.

Symptoms

- Chronic, bilateral ocular irritation, redness, burning, tearing, crusting

Signs

Skin Chronic hyperemia, telangiectasias, papules, pustules of nose, forehead and cheeks. Rhinophyma in advanced stages, especially in men (Figure 1-19A)

Eye Blepharitis, meibomitis, eyelid margin telangiectasias, recurrent chalazia, conjunctival or episcleral injection (Figure 1-19B).

Superficial punctate keratopathy, peripheral corneal vascularization, sterile marginal infiltrates, phlyctenules, peripheral corneal scarring, pannus, thinning, and occasionally corneal melting and perforation (Figure 1-19C)

Treatment

- Warm compresses 5 to 10 minutes bid and eyelid hygiene for blepharitis/meibomitis
- Minimally preserved or preservative-free artificial tears for dry eyes
- Judicious topical corticosteroid for sterile keratitis. When in doubt, treat an infiltrate as infectious keratitis.
- Topical tetracycline, bacitracin, or erythromycin ointment bid or qhs
- Oral tetracycline or erythromycin 250 mg qid or doxycycline 100 mg bid for 1 week, then half dose for 4 to 6 weeks. Can taper down to a minimum dosage (e.g., doxycycline 20 mg bid) for long-term treatment.
- Consider a dermatology consult if there is significant skin involvement.

Prognosis

- Good for improvement in symptoms, poor for total resolution of symptoms. Patients must realize rosacea is a chronic condition that can be effectively treated in most cases but not "cured."

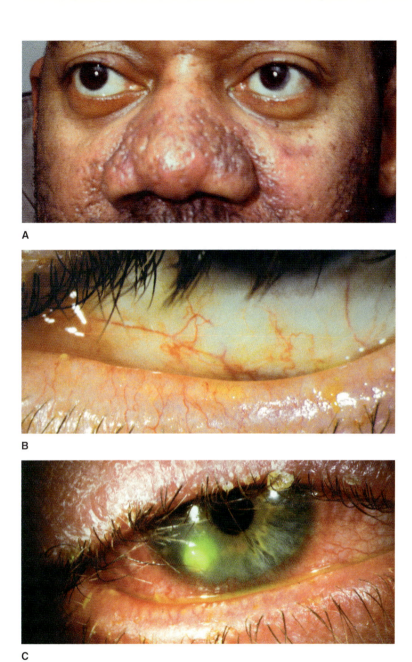

Figure 1-19   Ocular rosacea   A. *There are significant papules and pustules of the cheeks, nose, and eyebrow areas. Rhinophyma is apparent. Note the peripheral corneal scarring inferotemporally on the left from previous corneal infiltrate and melting.* **B.** *There are severe telangiectasias of the eyelid margin which is noticeably thickened. No patent meibomian gland orifices are visible.* **C.** *Telangiectasia and thickening of the eyelid margin, along with crusting of the eyelashes are seen in this patient with severe ocular rosacea. Diffuse conjunctival injection and a dense corneal scar from previous rosacea-related ulceration at the 7 o'clock position are present.*

Chapter 2

CONJUNCTIVAL DEGENERATIONS AND MASS LESIONS

PINGUECULA AND PTERYGIUM

Pingueculae and pterygia are extremely common conjunctival/corneal degenerations typically affecting patients living in equatorial regions where there is high exposure to sunlight.

Etiology

- Ultraviolet exposure
- Chronic dryness and hot, dusty environment
- These factors lead to elastotic degeneration of the substantia propria of the conjunctiva, resulting in subepithelial proliferation of fibrovascular tissue, initially on the conjunctiva and then on the cornea.

Symptoms

- Irritation, redness nasally or temporally, tearing, occasionally decreased vision

Signs

Pinguecula Yellow-white, often triangular, slightly elevated conjunctival lesion adjacent to the nasal or temporal side of the limbus (Figure 2-1A)

Pterygium Triangular, wing-shaped fibrovascular sheet of tissue extending onto the cornea at the 3 and 9 o'clock positions (Figure 2-1b). An iron line (Stocker's line) in the corneal epithelium may be present central to the apex of the pterygium.

- An area of thinning due to desiccation (delle) may be present in the cornea adjacent to an elevated lesion.

Differential Diagnosis

Pseudopterygium An adhesion of conjunctiva onto the corneal surface after corneal injury. Unlike a true pterygium, the adhesion is only at the apex and not throughout the underlying surface. It is typically unilateral and often not at the 3 and 9 o'clock positions.

Fuchs' Marginal Keratitis Associated with mild to severe peripheral corneal thinning

Conjunctival Papilloma, Nevus, Intraepithelial Neoplasia, or Squamous Cell Carcinoma If not typical for a pterygium or pinguecula, consider a conjunctival biopsy.

Diagnosis

- Slit-lamp examination to look for unusual features suspicious of other diagnoses. Pingueculae and pterygia have classic appearances.
- Excisional biopsy in cases suspicious of malignancy

Treatment

- Avoid excessive sunlight exposure and wear good ultraviolet blocking sunglasses.
- Artificial tears to prevent dry eyes
- Topical antihistamines (e.g., emedastine, levocabastine, antazoline, naphazoline), non-steroidal anti-inflammatory agents (e.g., ketoro-lac), or rarely corticosteroids (e.g., loteprednol 0.2%, fluorometholone 0.1%) bid to qid to reduce redness or inflammation
- Surgical excision is indicated if there is excessive irritation, difficulty with contact lens wear, for cosmetic reasons, or when there is progression towards the visual axis. The recurrence rate is much lower when excision is combined with a conjunctival autograft.
- Intraoperative application of mitomycin C and postoperative use of beta radiation may decrease the recurrence rate, but are associated with an increased risk of corneoscleral necrosis and are usually not necessary when a conjunctival autograft is performed.

Prognosis

Good to very good depending on severity. Pterygia can recur in about 10% to 15% of patients, occasionally worse than the original case.

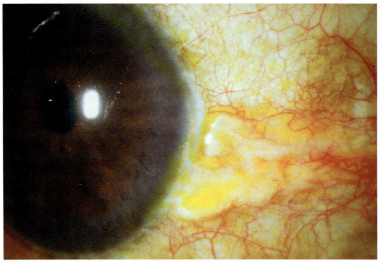

A

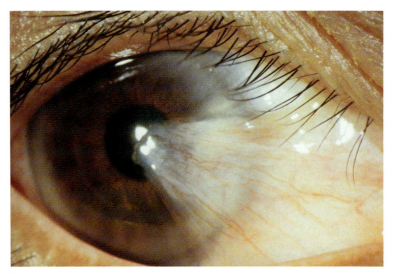

B

Figure 2-1   Pinguecula   **A.** *A triangular, creamy white elevated conjunctival mass is seen at the limbus from the 3 to 4 o'clock positions.* **Pterygium**   **B.** *A nasal wing-shaped fibrovascular growth is apparent in this patient's right eye with a classic nasal pterygium. This pterygium is reaching into the visual axis.*

OTHER CONJUNCTIVAL DEGENERATIONS

Amyloidosis

- Amyloidosis is a degenerative condition in which the noncollagenous protein amyloid is deposited in the conjunctiva (Figure 2-2A).
- It may be primary or secondary.
- It may be localized to the conjunctiva or be related to a systemic disorder.
- Primary localized amyloidosis is the most common form. Primary systemic amyloidosis involves amyloid deposition throughout the eye and eyelids and can affect the heart and kidneys.
- Rule out systemic amyloid conditions.

Calcium Concretions

- Calcium concretions are yellow-white calcium deposits that are embedded in the upper and/or lower palpebral conjunctiva.
- Generally they are located below the surface of the conjunctiva and do not cause any symptoms. Occasionally, the concretions erode through the surface of the conjunctiva, stain with fluorescein dye, and cause foreign body symptoms (Figure 2-2B).
- If mild, the symptoms can be treated with topical lubrication; if severe, the concretions can be removed but often recur.

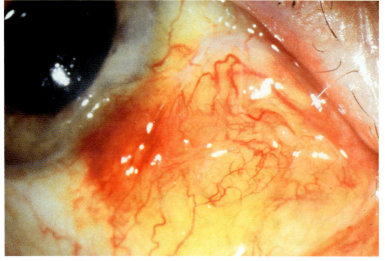

A

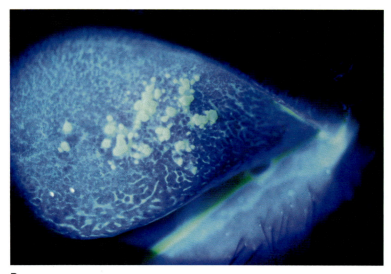

B

Figure 2-2 Conjunctival amyloidosis A. *An elevated yellow colored conjunctival mass is noted in this elderly patient. It was mobile over the sclera, and it did not have the classic appearance of a pterygium or the papillomatous pattern of a squamous cell tumor. Conjunctival biopsy revealed amyloidosis.* **Conjunctival calcium concretions B.** *Multiple white calcium concretions have eroded through the conjunctival epithelial surface of the upper eyelid, seen on eyelid eversion. These exposed concretions cause a chronic foreign body sensation and require removal.*

MELANOCYTIC CONJUNCTIVAL LESIONS

Conjunctival Epithelial Melanosis (Racial Melanosis)

- Common in pigmented races, usually bilateral, may have asymmetric ocular involvement, becomes more pronounced during puberty.
- Flat, patchy, brownish pigmentation scattered over the conjunctiva, but frequently involves the perilimbal regions (Figure 2-3A).
- Mobile over the sclera. May be perforated by anterior ciliary arteries or nerves.
- No malignant potential.

Oculodermal Melanosis (Nevus of Ota)

- A congenital condition characterized by blue-gray hyperpigmentation of skin and mucous membranes in the distribution of the fifth cranial nerve.
- Almost always unilateral.
- Three variants are seen: dermal, ocular, and oculodermal melanoses.
- Involves the dermis of the skin and episclera of the eye, thus the lesion does not move over the sclera.
- May affect ipsilateral uveal tissues, orbit, and central nervous system.
- Malignant transformation, uveal melanoma, and glaucoma can develop and patients should be followed-up regularly.

Nevus

- Develops during puberty or early adulthood.
- Most are subepithelial or compound nevi.
- Appears as a well-demarcated, flat or slightly elevated lesion, usually in the interpalpebral areas. It is usually solitary, and has a predilection for the limbus, plica, caruncle, and eyelid margin. Cystic spaces within the nevus are common and are the key to diagnosis. The degree of pigmentation may vary and may increase at puberty (Figure 2-3B).

- Enlargement can occur but may be a sign of malignant transformation. Nevi involving the cornea, tarsal or forniceal conjunctivae are extremely rare and should be excised for histopathologic evaluation.
- Periodic photographic documentation of the lesion may be helpful for follow-up.

Primary Acquired Melanosis

- This is a rare, unilateral, premalignant condition that is usually seen in elderly white patients.
- Unifocal or multifocal flat patches with indistinct margins that may involve any part of the conjunctiva. Cystic spaces are absent (Figure 2-3C).
- Follow-up with clinical documentation (e.g., slit-lamp photography) should be performed every 6 months. Malignant change should be suspected if the patches become nodular.
- Local wide excision with cryotherapy should be done for suspicious lesions. Incomplete excision and/or recurrence is common, requiring more aggressive treatment (e.g., local radiation therapy).

Secondary Acquired Melanosis

Causes are:

- Adrenochrome deposits: discrete clumps of melanin on tarsal and forniceal conjunctiva associated with long-term use of topical epinephrine
- Alkaptonuria: interpalpebral, bluish-gray or black pigmentation of the conjunctiva, episclera, sclera, and tendons of horizontal rectus muscles due to accumulation of homogentisic acid
- Mascara deposits
- Age-related
- Addison's disease
- Hemochromatosis
- Argyrosis: as a result of long-term use of drops containing silver
- Dark foreign bodies

Malignant Melanoma

- Malignant melanoma is an uncommon, malignant tumor that may be pigmented or nonpigmented. It may arise *de novo,* from preexisting primary acquired melanosis, or from a nevus.
- Elevated nodule that can affect any part of the conjunctiva, but has a predilection for the limbus and may extend onto the cornea. Feeder vessels may be seen (Figures 2-3D,E). Advanced melanomas may invade the eyelids and orbit.
- Treatment is local excision with cryotherapy. Local radiation therapy may also be beneficial. Exenteration may be necessary for orbital involvement. Use palliation with chemotherapy if metastasis is present (lymph nodes, central nervous system, liver, etc.).

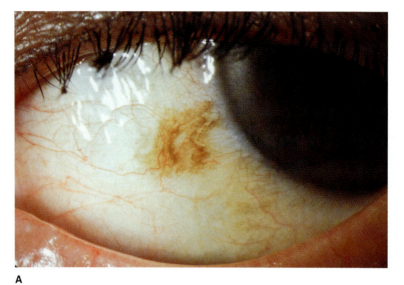

A

Figure 2-3   Conjunctival epithelial (racial) melanosis   A. *An area of poorly demarcated conjunctival epithelial melanin pigment is seen in this African American patient. These lesions have minimal to no malignant potential. (Continued.)*

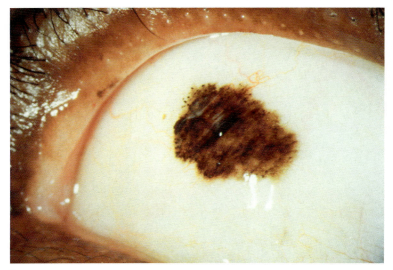

B

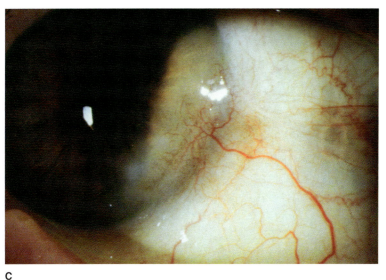

C

Figure 2-3 (cont.)   Conjunctival nevus   B. *A pigmented patch can be seen in the superior conjunctiva of this African American woman. It is well demarcated, has not changed in size, and has numerous microcysts, all pointing to the diagnosis of a nevus.* **Primary acquired melanosis   C.** *An area of flat conjunctival pigmentation is seen at the limbus from the 3 to 5 o'clock positions. There is a mild increase in vascularization. This lesion is suspicious for malignant transformation. (Continued.)*

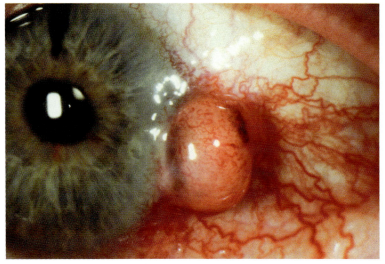

D

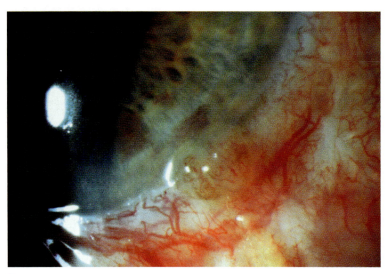

E

Figure 2-3 (cont.)   Malignant melanoma of the conjunctiva   D. *Biopsy of this large, solid conjunctival mass revealed malignant melanoma. It is relatively amelanotic, but pigmented areas can be seen at the 3 and 9 o'clock aspects of the lesion. There is also significant surrounding vascularization, indicating an aggressive process.* **E.** *A small recurrent conjunctival malignant melanoma is seen at the limbus at the 5 o'clock position after surgical excision. It was reexcised and treated with a radioactive plaque.*

BENIGN AMELANOCYTIC CONJUNCTIVAL LESIONS

Granulomas

Chalazion   Single nodule on the tarsal conjunctiva (see Figures 1-2A,B).

Pyogenic Granuloma   Vascularized nodule(s) of the bulbar or palpebral conjunctiva. They most commonly occur after conjunctival injury such as surgery or a chalazion (Figure 2-4A).

Sarcoidosis   Multiple yellow-colored nodules involving the tarsal or forniceal conjunctiva (Figure 2-4B). When present, biopsy can confirm the diagnosis of sarcoidosis.

Rhinosporidiosis   Very rare fungal infection that may cause conjunctival granulomas.

Vasculitides (e.g., Polyarteritis Nodosa, Churg-Strauss Syndrome)   Very friable lesions.

Epibulbar Dermoid

- Epibulbar dermoid is an uncommon, congenital lesion which may occur in isolation or in association with other ocular or systemic anomalies. May be unilateral or bilateral.
- Solid, smooth, round white mass typically located at the limbus, but may be elsewhere, even the central cornea. Lesions may encroach onto the cornea causing astigmatism. May have hair follicles (Figures 2-4C,D,E).
- Surgical resection may result in corneoscleral thinning and may have to be combined with a corneal lamellar patch graft or rarely a penetrating graft.

Ocular Associations   Eyelid coloboma, ocular coloboma.

Systemic Associations   Goldenhar's syndrome, most common, often bilateral dermoids; Treacher Collins syndrome; Franceschetti syndrome.

Lipodermoid

- A lipodermoid is an uncommon and often bilateral condition, typically found in adults.
- Large, yellow, soft, movable, subconjunctival lesions consisting of adipose and dermal tissues most commonly located superotemporally. Hair follicles may be seen on the surface. The lesions extend into the superior fornices, and it is impossible to visualize their posterior limits. Complete surgical excision is unnecessary and should be avoided to prevent damage to the rectus muscle, lacrimal gland, and the levator muscle.

Hereditary Benign Intraepithelial Dyskeratosis (HBID)

- HBID is a rare disorder characterized by marked conjunctival and episcleral vessel injection with overlying white plaques of acanthotic and dyskeratotic epithelial cells (Figure 2-4F).
- It is located primarily in the nasal and temporal interpalpebral zones.
- It is most commonly found in members of the Haliwa Indian tribes of North Carolina.
- No good treatment exists currently, although occasionally a conjunctival biopsy is required to rule out a conjunctival tumor.

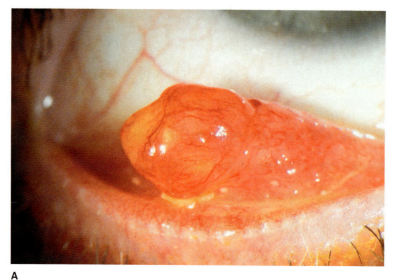

A

B

Figure 2-4 Pyogenic granuloma A. *This large collection of granulation tissue occurred as an inflammatory response after a inferior eyelid chalazion resolved.* **Sarcoid granulomas B.** *Multiple yellowish nodules are seen in the upper bulbar conjunctiva in this patient with sarcoidosis. In patients with suspected sarcoidosis and a conjunctival nodule, the diagnosis of sarcoidosis can often be confirmed with a simple conjunctival biopsy. (Continued.)*

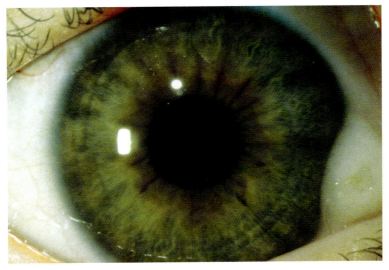

C

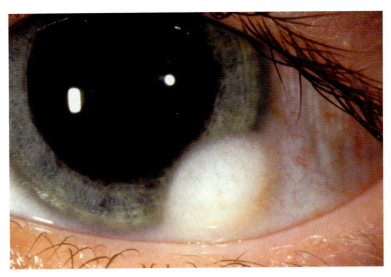

D

Figure 2-4 (cont.) **Epibulbar dermoid** *C. A large temporal solid limbal dermoid is seen. Note the cilia arising from the dermoid.* **Epibulbar dermoid** *D. An inferonasal dermoid can be seen in this 7-year-old girl. While her uncorrected vision was 20/20, she was very unhappy with its cosmetic appearance. (Continued.)*

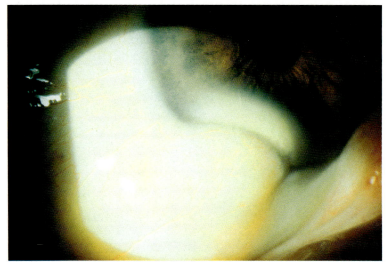

E

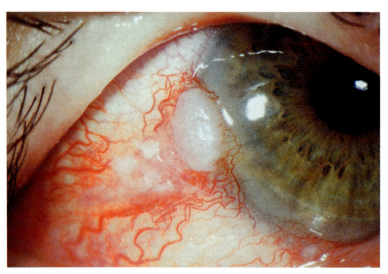

F

Figure 2-4 (cont.)   Epibulbar dermoid   E. *This inferotemporal dermoid encroaches on the cornea with secondary corneal scarring.* **Hereditary benign intraepithelial dyskeratosis (HBID)   F.** *Prominent conjunctival and episcleral injection with an overlying elevated white plaque is seen temporally in this right eye with HBID. The patient was quite photophobic.*

POTENTIALLY MALIGNANT AMELANOCYTIC CONJUNCTIVAL LESIONS

Squamous Papilloma

- Pedunculated squamous papilloma is an uncommon, benign tumor caused by the human papillomavirus. It typically occurs in children and young adults.
- Papillomas have fingerlike projections, and are located in the palpebral conjunctiva, fornix, or caruncle (Figure 2-5A). They may be multifocal or bilateral.
- They often resolve on their own. When large or chronic they can be excised but they may recur, occasionally worse than the original lesion. Application of cryotherapy at the base of the lesion after excision may decrease the risk of recurrence.
- A nonviral, sessile form that occurs in the elderly and involves the perilimbal conjunctiva is precancerous or cancerous and should be completely excised with wide margins and supplemental cryotherapy.

Conjunctival Intraepithelial Neoplasia

- Conjunctival intraepithelial neoplasia is a unilateral, premalignant condition that is seen in older, fair-skinned individuals. This condition was formerly referred to as Bowen's disease, intraepithelial epithelioma, and conjunctival dyskeratosis.
- The lesions are usually located at the limbus and may involve adjacent cornea (Figures 2-5B, C,D). The three clinical types are: (1) a fleshy gelatinous lesion with variable keratinization; (2) a white plaque (leukoplakic-type); and (3) papillary.
- Treatment is by complete surgical excision with supplemental cryotherapy.

Squamous Cell Carcinoma

- Invasive squamous cell carcinoma is a rare, slow-growing, locally invasive tumor which occurs most frequently at the limbus. It most

likely progresses from conjunctival intraepithelial neoplasia that breaks through the conjunctival basement membrane.
- Papillary or gelatinous tumor. Frequently associated with feeder blood vessels (Figure 2-5E).
- Treatment is by complete surgical excision with supplemental cryotherapy. A lamellar sclerectomy may be required to completely excise the lesion.
- Can be aggressive in immunocompromised patients.

Other Carcinomas

- Mucoepidermoid carcinoma and spindle cell carcinoma are similar to squamous cell carcinoma, but are more aggressive, and may arise anywhere on the conjunctiva.
- Sebaceous gland carcinoma is an uncommon and aggressive tumor that typically involves the upper eyelid of elderly patients, but may rarely arise *de novo* from the tarsal conjunctiva as a papillomatous or plaque-like lesion (Figure 2-5F). Can masquerade as chronic unilateral conjunctivitis or recurrent chalazia. May require multiple biopsies.

Reactive Lymphoid Hyperplasia and Non-Hodgkin's Lymphoma

- The appearance of the two conditions is similar.
- Smooth, fleshy, subconjunctival mass which may involve a large area (Figure 2-5G). The lesions may be single or multiple and involve both eyes in about 20% of cases. Small affected areas are called "salmon patches," and they occur most commonly in the bulbar or forniceal conjunctiva.
- Incisional or excisional biopsy should be performed and sent for immunohistochemical studies (which may require nonfixed tissue).
- A systemic evaluation should be performed by an internist or oncologist.

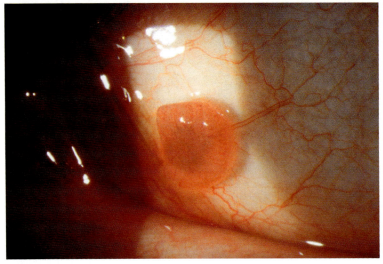

A

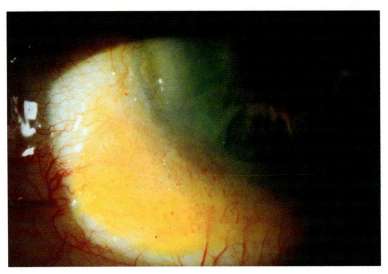

B

Figure 2-5   Conjunctival papilloma   A. *This squamous papilloma in a pediatric patient is likely of viral origin. It had numerous papillary vascular fronds attached to a stalk (pedunculated).* **Conjunctival intraepithelial neoplasia   B.** *Note the large, well-demarcated, sessile papillomatous lesion adjacent to the limbus from the 6 to 8 o'clock positions. Excisional biopsy revealed conjunctival intraepithelial neoplasia. (Continued.)*

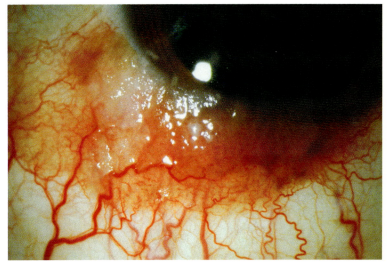

C

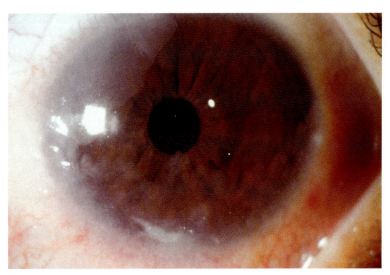

D

Figure 2-5 (cont.) Conjunctival intraepithelial neoplasia *C. This fleshy, sessile, mildly elevated mass lesion has a keratinized, leukoplakic component. Excisional biopsy revealed conjunctival intraepithelial neoplasia. D. This HIV-positive patient had a small limbal conjunctival lesion inferiorly. Thickened, gray-white fronds and sheets of abnormal epithelium is indicative of extensive corneal invasion from the 3 to 12 o'clock positions. (Continued.)*

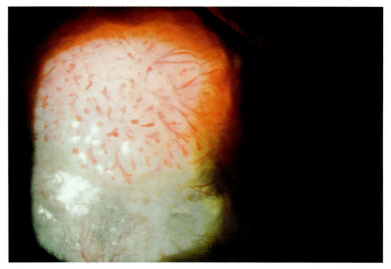

E

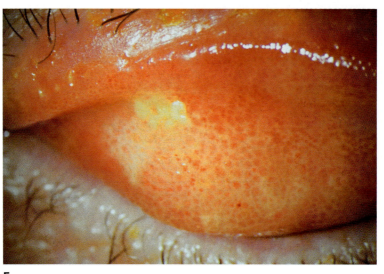

F

Figure 2-5 (cont.)   Squamous cell carcinoma   E. *A large, elevated conjunctival mass is seen at the superior limbus. The mass has vascularized papillomatous fronds. The lesion extends onto and covers most of the cornea. Conjunctival biopsy revealed squamous cell carcinoma.*
Sebaceous gland carcinoma   F. *The right upper eyelid is everted in this elderly patient with a chronic unilateral blepharoconjunctivitis demonstrating a diffuse thickened papillomatous conjunctival surface. Eyelid biopsy revealed sebaceous gland carcinoma. (Continued.)*

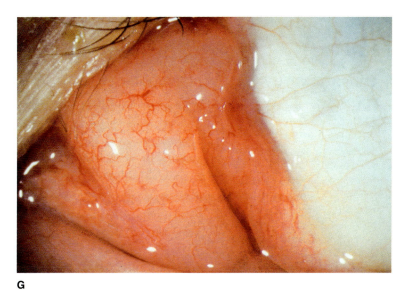

G

Figure 2-5 (cont.)   Conjunctival lymphoma   G. *This fleshy, salmon-colored mass adjacent to the caruncle was a conjunctival lymphoma. It was treated with surgical excision and local radiation treatment as work-up did not reveal evidence of systemic involvement.*

CYSTIC LESIONS

Primary Conjunctival Cyst

- A common, translucent cyst containing clear fluid on the bulbar conjunctiva. May be attached to the conjunctiva or freely mobile under the conjunctiva (Figure 2-6). Can cause a foreign body sensation.
- Differential diagnosis includes conjunctival lymphangiocele, which is often more tortuous.
- Treatment is usually unnecessary. If symptomatic, the cyst should be completely excised by shelling it out from under the conjunctiva. Puncturing the cyst with a needle or incomplete excision typically results in recurrence.

Iatrogenic Cysts

These cysts may take the following forms:

- Secondary implantation cysts following surgery or trauma.
- Drainage bleb following filtration surgery or blebs that may be flat and diffuse or localized after cataract surgery.
- Tenon's cyst associated with a filtration bleb, characterized by an elevated cystlike cavity with engorged surface vessels.

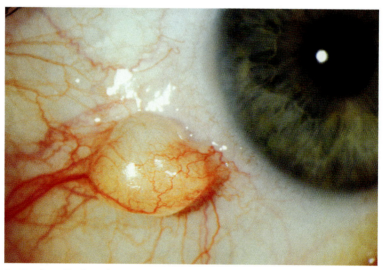

Figure 2-6 Conjunctival cyst *A large, mobile conjunctival cyst is seen near the limbus. It was large enough to cause chronic irritative symptoms. These can often be removed in toto by carefully incising the conjunctiva and gently shelling out the cyst.*

VASCULAR LESIONS

Telangiectasias

The following metabolic disorders may rarely be associated with dilated and tortuous blood vessels of the bulbar conjunctiva:

- Diabetes mellitus
- Fabry's disease: frequently associated with aneurysm formation
- Other metabolic disorders (e.g., fucosidosis, GM_1 gangliosidosis)
- Multiple endocrine neoplasia IIb: associated with prominent paralimbal nerve bundles

Hematologic Disorders

The following hematologic disorders may be associated with sludging of the blood:

- Dysproteinemias (e.g., multiple myeloma)
- Sickle cell anemia: isolated, corkscrew- or comma-shaped vessels
- Polycythemia vera

Hemorrhagic Lymphangiectasia

- Hemorrhagic lymphangiectasia is a rare condition that may occur after mild inflammation or trauma. It may also be associated with vascular malformations of the eyelid and parotid gland.
- Dilated and tortuous bulbar lymphatic vessels that may become filled with blood if they communicate with conjunctival veins.

Capillary Hemangioma

- Capillary hemangioma is an uncommon tumor that may be associated with hemangiomas of the eyelids and orbit.
- Bright red lesion that blanches with pressure. It may bleed spontaneously or following minor trauma.

Lymphangioma

- Lymphangioma is a rare tumor that may be associated with similar lesions of the orbit, face, sinuses, and oropharynx.
- Bright red lesion which is similar to, but may be larger than, a hemangioma.

Kaposi's Sarcoma

- Kaposi's sarcoma, occurring most commonly on the skin including the eyelids and occasionally on the conjunctiva, is often seen in AIDS patients.
- A reddish vascular conjunctival lesion that may be diffuse or nodular. A diffuse tumor may resemble a subconjunctival hemorrhage on cursory examination.
- No specific treatment is required. If severe, and systemic AIDS treatment and chemotherapy have been maximized, local excision, cryotherapy, or radiation can be used for ocular Kaposi's sarcoma.

Sturge-Weber Syndrome (Encephalotrigeminal Angiomatosis)

- Localized telangiectasias, probably associated with episcleral hemangiomas (Figure 2-7A).
- Look for glaucoma, iris hyperchromia, and diffuse choroidal hemangioma.

Carotid–Cavernous Sinus and Dural-Sinus Fistulas

- There are two types of arteriovenous fistulas that affect the eye. They produce reversal of flow through the superior ophthalmic vein that can be seen on color Doppler studies and dilation of the superior ophthalmic vein that can be seen on computed tomography or magnetic resonance imaging.

- A carotid–cavernous sinus fistula is a high-flow communication between the internal carotid artery and the cavernous sinus. It most commonly occurs after trauma or surgery but can arise spontaneously. It can produce severe conjunctival vessel engorgement and chemosis, eyelid swelling, pulsating exophthalmos, elevated intraocular pressure, and an orbital bruit.
- A dural-sinus fistula is a low-flow communication between the meningeal branches of the carotid artery and the cavernous sinus. They occur spontaneously, most commonly in middle-aged and elderly women. The clinical findings are much milder than in carotid–cavernous sinus fistulas, although the intraocular pressure can be quite elevated. The chronic red eye is often mistaken for chronic conjunctivitis (Figure 2-7B).
- Both forms can cause arterialization of the conjunctival blood vessels resulting in the characteristic corkscrew pattern.
- Treatment is with closure of the fistula through an endoarterial balloon embolization or surgery, although dural-sinus fistulas can close spontaneously or after angiography.

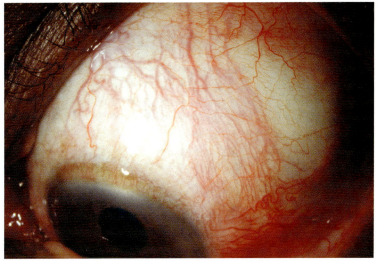

A

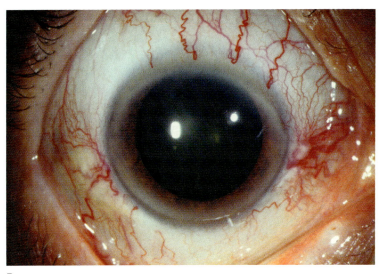

B

Figure 2-7 Sturge-Weber syndrome A. *Prominent episcleral vessels are seen superiorly in this patient with Sturge-Weber syndrome. Elevated episcleral venous pressure can cause glaucoma.* **Cavernous sinus fistula** B. *This patient had a low flow dural-sinus fistula. Note the engorged corkscrew episcleral vessels. The intraocular pressure was moderately elevated.*

Chapter 3

ANTERIOR SEGMENT DEVELOPMENTAL ANOMALIES

ANOMALIES OF CORNEAL SIZE AND SHAPE

MICROCORNEA

Microcornea is an uncommon congenital unilateral or bilateral condition. Inheritance is autosomal dominant or recessive.

Signs

- Infant horizontal corneal diameter less than 10 mm; adult horizontal corneal diameter less than 11 mm (Figure 3-1).
- Shallow anterior chamber, angle-closure or open-angle glaucoma, corneal flattening, and hyperopia.
- May have associated nanophthalmos (Table 3-1).
- Other ocular dimensions are normal.

Treatment

- Manage refractive error and search for other ocular and systemic anomalies.

Prognosis

- Varies depending on associated ocular and systemic abnormalities

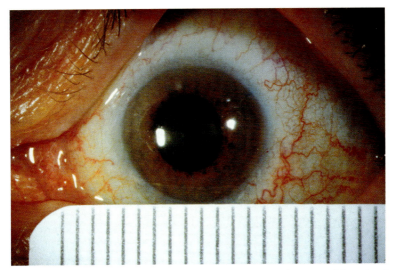

Figure 3-1 **Microcornea** *This cornea measured 8.5–9.0 mm in diameter. Otherwise the eye was essentially normal.*

TABLE 3-1 **ASSOCIATIONS OF MICROCORNEA**

Ocular	Systemic Syndromes
• Anterior segment dysgeneses	• Cornelia de Lange's
• Congenital cataract	• Ehlers-Danlos'
• Congenital glaucoma	• Nance-Horan
• Corneal leukoma	• Trisomy 13, 18, 21
• Cornea plana	• Turner's
• Hyperopia	• Waardenburg's
• Microphakia	• Weill-Marchesani
• Uveal coloboma	

MEGALOCORNEA

Megalocornea is an uncommon congenital, bilateral condition that is usually inherited in an X-linked recessive manner and is therefore mostly found in males.

Signs

- Clear cornea with a horizontal diameter of greater than 12 mm in the neonate and 13 mm in adults (Figure 3-2).
- Very deep anterior chamber.
- Normal intraocular pressure.
- Corneal steepening, high myopia, and astigmatism, but good visual acuity.
- Lens subluxation may occur as a result of zonular stretching.
- May develop glaucoma secondary to angle abnormalities.

Treatment

- Manage refractive error and search for other ocular and systemic anomalies, especially glaucoma and lens abnormalities.

Prognosis

- Generally good, but depends on associated ocular and systemic abnormalities (Table 3-2).

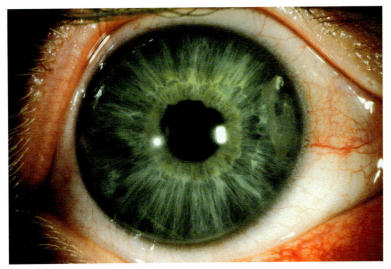

Figure 3-2 Megalocornea *This cornea measured 14 mm in diameter. The cornea is clear except for some calcific degeneration nasally and temporally.*

TABLE 3-2 ASSOCIATIONS OF MEGALOCORNEA

Ocular	Systemic Syndromes
• Astigmatism	• Albinism
• Axenfeld-Rieger anomaly	• Alport's
• Cataract	• Apert's
• Congenital glaucoma	• Craniosynostosis
• Ectopia lentis	• Down's
• Myopia	• Ehlers-Danlos'
	• Marfan's
	• Osteogenesis imperfecta
	• Progressive facial hemiatrophy

NANOPHTHALMOS

Nanophthalmos is an uncommon, congenital, bilateral condition in which the globe has reduced volume but is otherwise grossly normal.

Signs

- Very high hyperopia (e.g., +12D to +15D).
- Adult corneal diameter is reduced, but the lens has a normal volume.
- Short axial length (e.g., 16–18 mm).
- Shallow anterior chamber.
- Thick sclera.
- Fundus may show a crowded disc, vascular tortuosity, and macular hypoplasia.

Associated Problems

- Angle-closure glaucoma
- Uveal effusion
- Retinal detachment
- Poorly tolerated intraocular surgery

MICROPHTHALMOS

Microphthalmos is an uncommon unilateral or bilateral condition in which the axial length of the eye is reduced and the eye is malformed (Figure 3-3). The effects on vision depend on its severity and the presence of associated anomalies. There are two types of microphthalmos: noncolobomatous and colobomatous (Table 3-3).

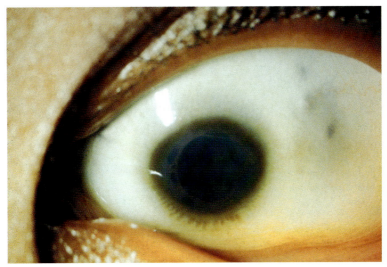

Figure 3-3   Microphthalmos   *This microphthalmic eye has a small cornea, abnormal iris, and overall small size. (Photo courtesy of Peter Laibson, MD.)*

TABLE 3-3   **TYPES OF MICROPHTHALMOS**

Noncolobomatous	Colobomatous
Isolated	Isolated
• Sporadic	• Sporadic
• Inherited (dominant, recessive, X-linked recessive)	• Inherited (dominant)
	With systemic syndromes:
With anterior persistent hyperplastic primary vitreous	• Patau's (trisomy 13)
	• Edward's (trisomy 18)
	• Cat-eye (partial trisomy 22)
Intrauterine infections (rubella, toxoplasmosis, cytomegalovirus, varicella)	• CHARGE
	• Meckel
	• Lenz microphthalmos

CHARGE syndrome is *c*oloboma, *h*eart anomaly, choanal *a*tresia, *r*etardation, and *g*enital or *e*ar anomalies.

BUPHTHALMOS

Buphthalmos is an uncommon, usually bilateral condition in which the globe is enlarged due to stretching of the cornea and sclera as a result of increased intraocular pressure before birth or during the first 3 years of life.

Signs

- Large cornea with variable scarring
- Horizontal or curvilinear ruptures in Descemet's membrane (Haab's striae) (Figure 3-4)
- Very deep anterior chamber
- Angle anomalies
- Myopia
- Optic disc cupping

Associations of Infantile Glaucoma

Ocular
- Aniridia
- Anterior segment dysgeneses
- Congenital ectropion uveae

Systemic
- Down's syndrome
- Lowe's syndrome
- Mucopolysaccharidoses
- Neurofibromatosis type 1
- Nevus of Ota
- Patau's syndrome (trisomy 13)
- Pierre Robin's syndrome
- Rieger's syndrome
- Sturge-Weber's syndrome

Treatment

- Management of glaucoma by a glaucoma specialist.

Prognosis

- Guarded, depending on amount of optic nerve damage prior to diagnosis, efficacy of treatment, and associated ocular and systemic disorders. Haab's striae of the cornea do not prevent good vision.

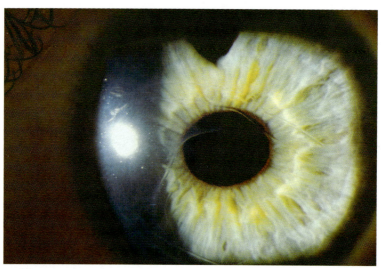

Figure 3-4 Haab's striae *These breaks in Descemet's membrane occurred secondary to congenital glaucoma. Note the multiple parallel swirling lines, which are rolled up edges of Descemet's membrane.*

CONGENITAL ANTERIOR STAPHYLOMA/KERATECTASIA

Congenital anterior staphyloma and keratectasia are extremely rare, congenital, usually unilateral conditions resulting in severe corneal protrusion and occasionally perforation (Figure 3-5).

Etiology

- It is probably due to intrauterine keratitis.

Signs

- Severe corneal opacification and protrusion of corneal tissue beyond the plane of the eyelids.
- Endothelium, Descemet's, and posterior corneal tissue are absent.
- It may be lined by uveal tissue posteriorly.

Treatment

- A penetrating keratoplasty can be attempted in bilateral cases. Most eyes will undergo an enucleation.

Prognosis

- Poor

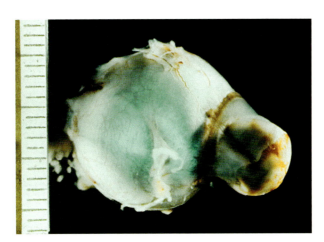

Figure 3-5   Keratectasia   *Gross specimen after enucleation of an eye with a large corneal staphyloma after suspected intrauterine infection. Note the massive protrusion anterior to the corneal limbus. (Photo courtesy of Peter Laibson, MD.)*

SCLEROCORNEA

Sclerocornea is a rare, congenital, usually bilateral nonprogressive, noninflammatory condition. It can be partial or complete.

Etiology

- Unknown.
- Most cases are sporadic.

Signs

- Opacification and vascularization of the peripheral or entire cornea. If only the peripheral cornea is involved, the resulting "scleralization" makes the cornea appear smaller than normal (Figures 3-6A,B).
- Often associated with cornea plana.
- May have associated glaucoma.

Ocular Associations

- Anterior segment dysgeneses
- Blue sclera
- Congenital cataract
- Cornea plana
- Glaucoma
- Iris abnormalities (e.g., aniridia, colohoma)
- Microphthalmos

Treatment

- If unilateral, may opt to follow the eye. If bilateral, consider a penetrating keratoplasty.

Prognosis

- Penetrating keratoplasty has a relatively poor prognosis in sclerocornea.

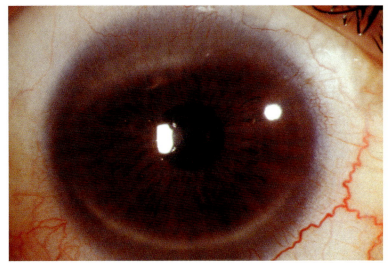

A

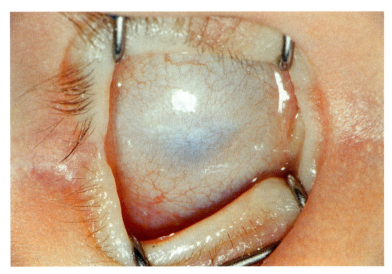

B

Figure 3-6   Peripheral sclerocornea   A. *The entire corneal periphery, but especially the superior and inferior cornea, are scleralized.* **Total sclerocornea   B.** *The entire cornea is scleralized. There is a slightly less opaque area centrally, which turned out to be the central cornea during penetrating keratoplasty.*

CORNEA PLANA

Cornea plana is a rare, congenital, bilateral condition. Many physicians consider it a mild form of sclerocornea.

Etiology

- Unknown

Symptoms

- None or poor vision

Signs

- Hyperopia
- Severe decrease in corneal curvature, where the sclera and cornea have the same curvature (Figure 3-7).
- Shallow anterior chamber
- Glaucoma

Ocular Associations

- Aniridia
- Anterior segment dysgeneses
- Microcornea
- Microphthalmos
- Sclerocornea

Treatment

- Correct refractive error. Contact lenses can be difficult to fit due to flatness of the cornea and the lack of difference between the corneal and scleral curvature.

Prognosis

- Good

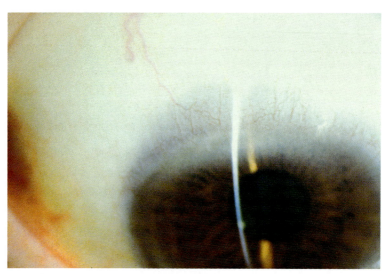

Figure 3-7 Peripheral sclerocornea/cornea plana *A slit-lamp view of the eye seen in Figure 3-6A demonstrates the lack of change in corneal curvature between the sclera and the cornea. The cornea had a flat corneal curvature and the eye was hyperopic.*

ANOMALIES OF THE ANTERIOR SEGMENT: ANTERIOR SEGMENT DYSGENESES

POSTERIOR EMBRYOTOXON

- Posterior embryotoxon is a creamy-white thickened, anteriorly displaced Schwalbe's line seen in the corneal periphery (Figure 3-8A).
- It is typically a bilateral condition that occurs to some extent in approximately 15% of normals. It is present in all patients with Axenfeld's and Rieger's anomaly.

AXENFELD'S ANOMALY

- Axenfeld's anomaly is a rare, bilateral, autosomal dominant or sporadic anomaly. It is characterized by strands of iris which span across the angle and attach to a posterior embryotoxon (Figure 3-8B).
- Glaucoma develops in 50% of cases, and the disorder is then known as Axenfeld's syndrome.

RIEGER'S ANOMALY

- Rieger's anomaly is a rare, bilateral, autosomal dominant or sporadic anomaly. It is characterized by posterior embryotoxon with adherent iris strands and iris stromal hypoplasia (Figure 3-8C). There may be pseudopolycoria, corectopia, and ectropion uveae.
- Of those affected, 50% of patients develop glaucoma.

RIEGER'S SYNDROME

- Autosomal dominant trait. Usually bilateral but asymmetric.
- Consists of Rieger's anomaly plus dental (hypodontia, microdontia) or facial (maxillary hypoplasia, telecanthus, hypertelorism) malformations.
- Of those affected, 50% of patients develop glaucoma.

PETERS' ANOMALY

- Sporadic inheritance, although autosomal recessive and dominant patterns have been reported.
- Bilateral in 80% of cases but asymmetric.
- Central corneal opacity, posterior Descemet's membrane or stromal defect, iridocorneal adhesions, possible lens-cornea adhesion and shallow anterior chamber (Figures 3-8D,E).
- May be associated with lens displacement and cataract.
- Of those affected, 50% of patients develop glaucoma.
- May have associated systemic abnormalities (e.g., skeletal, dental).

LOCALIZED POSTERIOR KERATOCONUS

- Very rare, sporadic, usually unilateral developmental anomaly presenting at birth.
- Nonprogressive protrusion of central area of the posterior corneal surface (Figure 3-8F).
- May have a mild corneal scar.
- Myopic astigmatism can occur.

DIAGNOSIS OF ANTERIOR SEGMENT ANOMALIES

- Family history for similar condition and systemic history for associated anomalies.
- Examine under anesthesia if unable to do an adequate evaluation in the office, including a slit-lamp examination, measurement of corneal diameter, intraocular pressure, gonioscopy, ophthalmoscopy, and retinoscopy. Ultrasound biomicroscopy can be helpful in imaging the anterior segment and B-scan ultrasonography can be used to image the posterior segment when necessary.

TREATMENT OF ANTERIOR SEGMENT ANOMALIES

- Visual rehabilitation: correct refractive errors, treat amblyopia, control glaucoma with medications or surgery, cataract extraction and corneal transplant as necessary. May need combined efforts of specialists in cornea, glaucoma, retinal, and pediatric ophthalmology.
- Refer to a pediatrician for management of systemic abnormalities.
- Chromosomal analysis and genetic counseling.

PROGNOSIS FOR ANTERIOR SEGMENT ANOMALIES

- Excellent for posterior embryotoxon and localized posterior keratoconus; fair to good for Axenfeld's and Rieger's anomalies; guarded for Peters' anomaly. The prognosis depends greatly on the severity of the glaucoma. Eyes with Peters' anomaly can do well with corneal transplantation; the success rate is worse when the lens is involved.

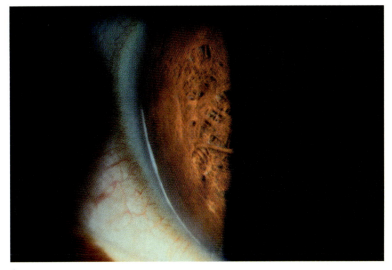

A

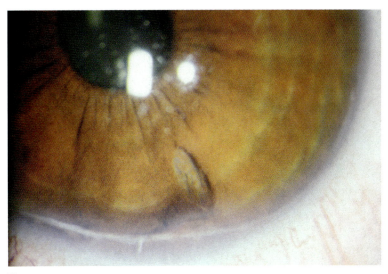

B

Figure 3-8 **Posterior embryotoxon** A. *A prominent Schwalbe's line can be seen from the 7 o'clock to the 9 o'clock positions. (Photo courtesy of Irving Raber, MD.)* **Axenfeld's anomaly** B. *A prominent Schwalbe's ring with iris adhesions can be seen inferiorly in this eye with Axenfeld's anomaly. (Photo courtesy of Elisabeth Cohen, MD.) (Continued.)*

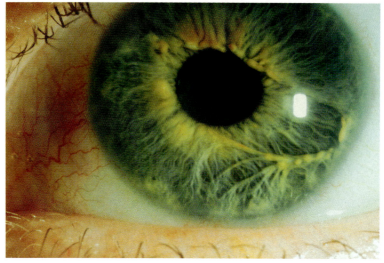

C

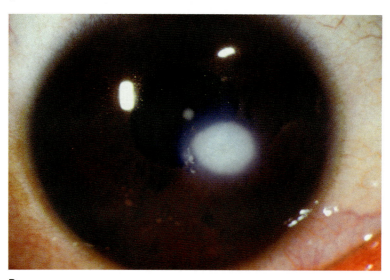

D

Figure 3-8 (cont.) Rieger's anomaly *C. A prominent Schwalbe's ring is present nasally and temporally in this eye with Rieger's anomaly. There is iris atrophy with mild corectopia temporally. (Photo courtesy of Peter Laibson, MD.)* **Peters' anomaly** *D. This eye with Peters' anomaly has a dense paracentral corneal opacity. There is a band of iris from the 3 o'clock pupillary margin to the corneal opacity. (Continued.)*

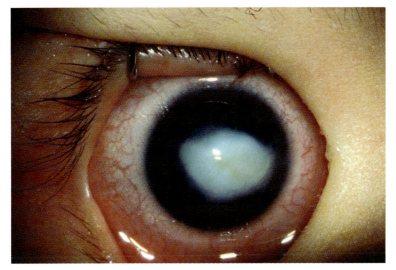

E

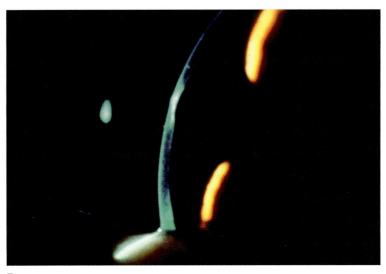

F

Figure 3-8 (cont.)   Peters' anomaly   E. *This dense central corneal opacity was associated with iris adhesions from the pupillary margin to the posterior aspect of the corneal opacity in this 4-year-old girl born in China. Her other eye had a similar condition requiring corneal transplants in both eyes.* **Posterior keratoconus   F.** *An indentation of the posterior cornea can be seen centrally which is characteristic of posterior keratoconus. There is a mild associated corneal opacity. There is minimal anterior corneal change, but there may be astigmatism.*

ANIRIDIA

Aniridia is a rare, bilateral condition which is associated with glaucoma in 75% of cases. Two thirds of patients have an autosomal dominant form which is not associated with Wilms' tumor. Approximately one third of cases are sporadic; 25% of sporadic cases will develop Wilms' tumor.

Signs

- Partial or essentially complete absence of the iris.
- Synechial angle-closure glaucoma occurs in 75% of cases as a result of pulling forward of rudimentary iris tissue.
- Associated ocular and systemic disorders.

Classification of Aniridia

- AN-1: Isolated (autosomal dominant): vision is poor due to foveal hypoplasia.
- AN-2: Isolated (autosomal dominant): vision is normal.
- AN-3 (Gillespie's syndrome): autosomal recessive. Mental handicap, cerebellar ataxia.
- AN-4 (Miller's syndrome): deletion of the short arm of chromosome 11, sporadic. Wilms' tumor, genitourinary anomalies, mental retardation.
- AN-5: variable inheritance. Iris hypoplasia with other ocular malformations (e.g., Peters' anomaly, microcornea, congenital aphakia, ectopia lentis).
- AN-6: variable inheritance. Iris hypoplasia with other systemic syndromes (e.g., Beimond's syndrome, absence of patella).

Ocular Associations of Aniridia

- Glaucoma
- Corneal lesions: pannus, opacity (Figure 3-9), keratolenticular adhesions, microcornea, sclerocornea
- Lens and iris changes: congenital aphakia, anterior polar, posterior subcapsular cataract, subluxation, ectopia lentis, persistent pupillary membranes
- Fundus lesions: foveal hypoplasia, disc hypoplasia, colobomas
- Nystagmus

Diagnosis

- Family history for similar condition and systemic history for associated anomalies.
- Examine under anesthesia if unable to do an adequate evaluation in the office, including a slit-lamp examination, measurement of corneal diameter and intraocular pressure, gonioscopy, ophthalmoscopy, and retinoscopy.

Treatment

- Visual rehabilitation: Correct refractive errors, treat amblyopia, and control glaucoma with medications or surgery. Cataract extraction and corneal transplant/limbal stem cell transplant as necessary.
- Chromosomal analysis and genetic counseling.
- Renal evaluation by pediatrician or pediatric oncologist to monitor for Wilms' tumor.

Prognosis

- Fair, depending on severity of glaucoma and corneal abnormalities. The limbal stem cell abnormality often leads to corneal haze and scarring. Corneal transplants often fail due to limbal stem cell deficiency. Limbal stem cell transplants with chronic systemic immunosuppression has a reasonably good prognosis.

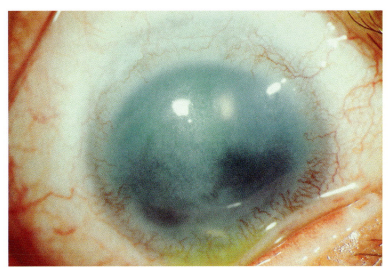

Figure 3-9   Aniridia   *This eye with aniridia demonstrates corneal pannus and severe corneal scarring. While there is a hazy view, no iris was present on slit-lamp examination.*

IRIS COLOBOMA

Iris coloboma is an uncommon, unilateral or bilateral condition caused by defective closure of the embryonic fissure, usually inferonasally. Isolated iris colobomas are either sporadic or dominantly inherited.

Signs

- A total coloboma is a segmental absence of iris from pupil to root, giving rise to a "keyhole" pupil.
- A partial coloboma does not involve the iris root (Figure 3-10).

Ocular Associations

- Colobomas of the ciliary body, lens, retina, choroid, and optic nerve
- Microphthalmos

Systemic Associations

- Cat-eye syndrome (partial trisomy 22)
- CHARGE syndrome (*c*oloboma, *h*eart anomaly, choanal *a*tresia, *r*etardation, and *g*enital or *e*ar anomalies)
- Edward's syndrome (trisomy 18)
- Patau's syndrome (trisomy 13)
- Rubinstein-Taybi's syndrome

Diagnosis

- Family history for similar condition and systemic history for associated anomalies.
- Examine under anesthesia if unable to do an adequate evaluation in the office, including a slit-lamp examination, measurement of corneal diameter and intraocular pressure, gonioscopy, ophthalmoscopy and retinoscopy. Ultrasound biomicroscopy can be helpful in imaging the anterior segment and B-scan ultrasonography can be used to image the posterior segment when necessary.

Treatment

- Manage refractive error and search for other anterior and posterior segment anomalies.
- Chromosomal analysis and genetic counseling.

Prognosis

- Depends on severity of the coloboma and on the extent of other ocular and systemic abnormalities.

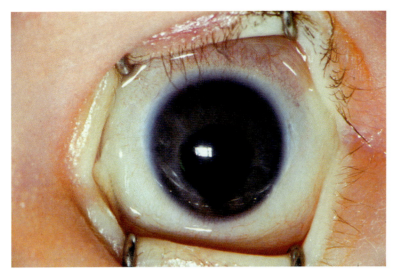

Figure 3-10 Iris coloboma *An inferior iris coloboma is present in this newborn with numerous systemic abnormalities. There are fine iris strands inferiorly. The other eye, which had severe sclerocornea, is seen in Figure 3-6B.*

Chapter 4

ECTATIC CONDITIONS OF THE CORNEA

KERATOCONUS

Keratoconus is a fairly common condition characterized by corneal thinning, protrusion, and irregularity. It is usually bilateral, although the severity of involvement may be asymmetric.

Etiology

- Sporadic or autosomal dominant with incomplete penetrance

Symptoms

- Gradually decreasing vision, beginning in adolescence and progressing into adult life.
- Patients often relate a history of not being able to attain good vision despite multiple changes of glasses or soft contact lenses.
- May have a history of eye rubbing.
- Can develop acutely decreased vision and pain due to hydrops with advanced disease.

Signs

Early
- Progressive myopia and astigmatism
- Scissors reflex on retinoscopy
- Irregular mires on keratometry
- Inferior steepening on computerized corneal topography (Figure 4-1A)
- Central or paracentral stromal thinning of the cornea with protrusion at the apex of the thinning (Figure 4-1B)
- Fleischer's ring: epithelial iron deposits at the base of the cone (Figure 4-1C)
- Prominent corneal nerves (Figure 4-1D)

Late
- Vogt's striae: fine vertical deep stromal tension lines which temporarily disappear with digital pressure applied to the limbus (Figure 4-1E)
- Abnormal "oil droplet" red reflex
- Rizutti's sign: conical light reflection on the nasal limbus when light is shone from the temporal side
- Variable corneal scarring, depending on severity (Figure 4-1F). May develop an elevated apical nodule (Figure 4-1G)
- Munson's sign: bulging of the lower eyelid in downgaze
- Acute hydrops: severe corneal edema resulting from a tear in Descemet's membrane (Figures 4-1H,I)

Associations of Keratoconus

Ocular Vernal disease, blue sclera, retinitis pigmentosa, Leber's congenital amaurosis

Systemic Down's syndrome, Ehlers-Danlos' syndrome, Apert's syndrome, ocular allergies, osteogenesis imperfecta

Differential Diagnosis

- Pellucid marginal degeneration: inferior peripheral corneal thinning with protrusion of the cornea above the area of maximal thinning

Treatment

Mild Cases   Glasses and soft contact lenses.

Moderate Cases   Rigid gas-permeable contact lens (RGPCL) or a hybrid lens.

Severe and Contact Lens-Intolerant Cases
- Penetrating keratoplasty.
- Refractive surgery in patients with keratoconus is unpredictable and generally not recommended.

- Lamellar keratoplasty, deep anterior lamellar keratoplasty, epikeratoplasty, and thermokeratoplasty are rarely performed.

Prognosis

- Most patients do well with RGPCLs. The success rate with corneal transplantation in keratoconus is high.

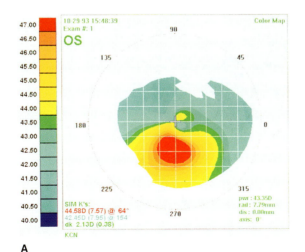

A

Figure 4-1   Keratoconus corneal topography   **A.** *Significant inferior corneal steepening is apparent using computerized corneal topographic analysis in this eye with moderate keratoconus. As seen on the color scale on the left, the red colors indicate corneal steepening and blue colors indicate corneal flattening. (Continued.)*

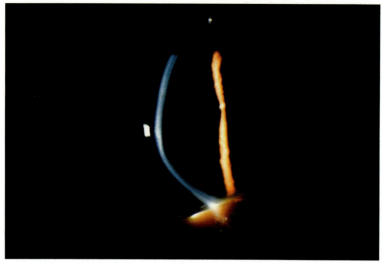

B

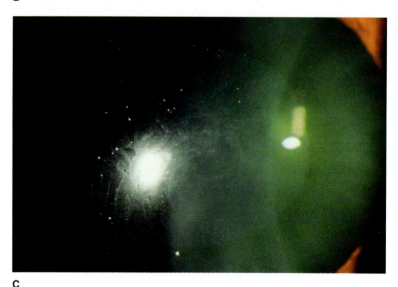

C

Figure 4-1 (cont.) Keratoconus *B. Slit-lamp view of this eye with significant keratoconus demonstrates inferocentral corneal thinning and steepening. Note the thinnest and most protruded areas of cornea coincide.* *C. A prominent Fleischer's ring, iron pigment deposition at the base of the cone, is present in this eye with keratoconus. (Continued.)*

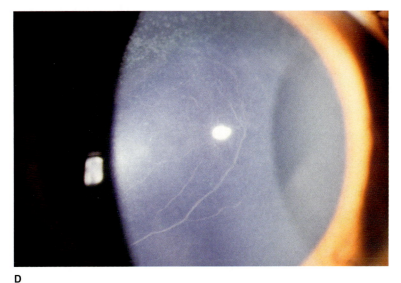

D

E

Figure 4-1 (cont.)   Keratoconus   D. *Prominent corneal nerves can be seen in this eye with keratoconus. These nerves can be distinguished from corneal "ghost" blood vessels as "ghost" vessels have a lumen, making them appear as two parallel lines.* **E.** *Faint, vertical posterior stromal stress lines, Vogt's striae, are visible at the apex of the cone. Gentle pressure on the limbus can cause these lines to change direction or disappear. (Continued.)*

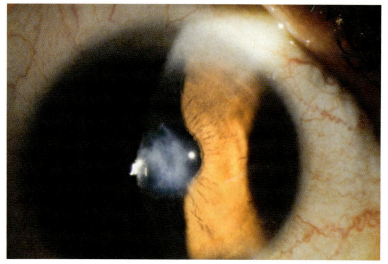

F

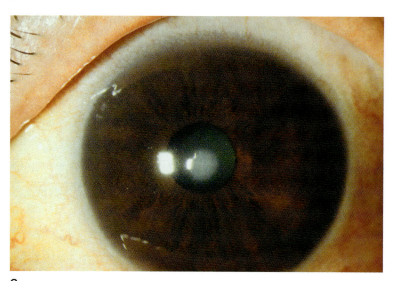

G

Figure 4-1 (cont.)   Keratoconus   F. *Significant central stromal scarring is present in this eye with advanced keratoconus.* **G.** *A hypertrophic nodule is present at the apex of the cone. These nodules can occur de novo or as a result of rigid contact lens wear. Such a nodule can affect vision and/or interfere with comfortable contact lens wear. These nodules can be removed with a superficial keratectomy or excimer laser phototherapeutic keratectomy (PTK). (Continued.)*

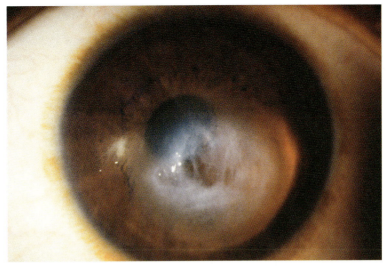

H

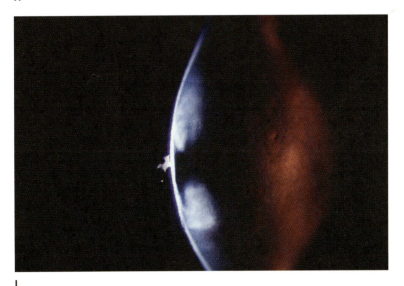

I

Figure 4-1 (cont.)   Keratoconus   H. *Acute corneal hydrops occurs when the cornea stretches to such a degree that a tear develops in Descemet's membrane, allowing inflow of aqueous fluid into the corneal stroma. The corneal stroma can swell to greater than five times its normal thickness. Acute hydrops is associated with a sudden decrease in vision and increase in pain.* **I.** *Slit-lamp view of the cornea seen in Figure 4-1H. Note the severe corneal thickening. A prominent cleft is apparent centrally, where corneal lamellae are separated by a large degree of aqueous fluid.*

PELLUCID MARGINAL DEGENERATION

Pellucid marginal degeneration is an uncommon, bilateral condition with inferior corneal thinning, protrusion, and irregularity. It usually presents in early adulthood.

Etiology

- Sporadic

Symptoms

- Gradually decreasing vision beginning in young adulthood. Can develop acute decreased vision and pain due to hydrops with advanced disease.

Signs

- High irregular against-the-rule astigmatism (flat at 90 degrees, steep at 180 degrees).
- Recognizable pattern of irregular astigmatism on computerized corneal topography (Figure 4-2A).
- Inferior, crescent-shaped band of peripheral corneal thinning, 1 to 2 mm in width, extending from the 4 o'clock to the 8 o'clock position, which is separated from the limbus by normal cornea (Figure 4-2B).
- The area of protrusion is located above the band of thinning (Figure 4-2C).
- Fleischer's ring and Vogt's striae are absent.
- Corneal hydrops occurs on rare occasion.

Differential Diagnosis

- Keratoconus: inferocentral corneal thinning with protrusion of cornea in the area of greatest thinning. A Fleischer's ring and Vogt's striae may be present.

Treatment

Mild and Moderate Cases RGPCL or a hybrid lens.

Severe and Contact Lens-Intolerant Cases
- Large inferior penetrating keratoplasty.
- Refractive surgery in patients with pellucid marginal degeneration is unpredictable and not recommended.
- Deep anterior lamellar keratoplasty and crescentic penetrating keratoplasty are occasionally performed.

Prognosis

- Most patients do well with RGPCLs, although they are harder to fit than keratoconus patients. The success rate with corneal transplantation in pellucid marginal degeneration is good, but not as good as keratoconus, due to more peripheral disease.

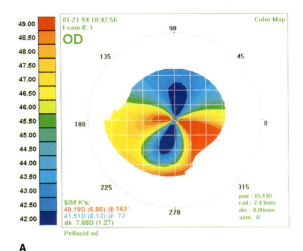

A

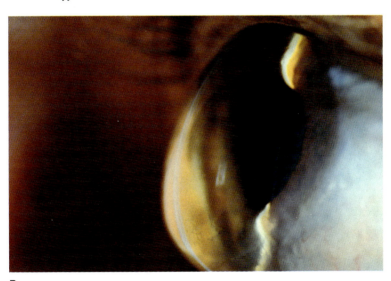

B

Figure 4-2 Pellucid marginal degeneration corneal topography A. *Significant irregular nasal and temporal corneal steepening is apparent in this computerized corneal topographic analysis of this eye with moderate pellucid marginal degeneration. Classically, the steepening is seen to curve around inferiorly in this condition. As seen on the color scale on the left, the red colors indicate corneal steepening and blue colors indicate corneal flattening.* **Pellucid marginal degeneration B.** *Side view demonstrates corneal protrusion inferiorly with significant steepening near the limbus. (Continued.)*

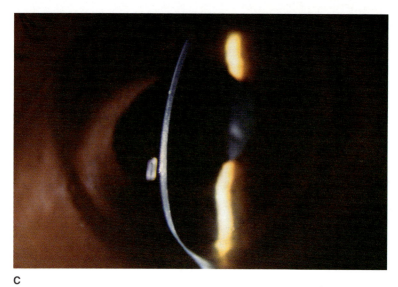

C

Figure 4-2 (cont.)   Pellucid marginal degeneration   **C.** *Slit-lamp view reveals corneal thinning approximately 2 mm from the inferior limbus. There is significant corneal steepening inferiorly. Note the most protruded portion of the cornea is above the thinnest area.*

KERATOGLOBUS

Keratoglobus is an extremely rare, bilateral condition of severe uniform peripheral corneal thinning. It usually presents at or shortly after birth.

Etiology

• Unknown

Symptoms

• Poor vision, occasionally pain due to hydrops

Signs

• Total corneal thinning with maximal thinning in the midperiphery, resulting in protrusion of the entire cornea (Figure 4-3A,B).
• The cornea can be very thin.
• Normal corneal diameter; very deep anterior chamber.
• Acute hydrops may occur in advanced cases.
• May develop a corneal perforation from minimal trauma because of the severe corneal thinning.

Systemic Associations

• A syndrome comprising blue sclera, hyperextensible joints, dental and hearing abnormalities
• Hyperthyroidism
• Rubinstein-Taybi syndrome

Treatment

• Mild and moderate cases: spectacles, which improve vision and provide some protection against trauma.
• Severe cases: some patients do well with a scleral contact lens.
• Surgical treatment is problematic. A large tectonic lamellar graft followed many months later by a smaller penetrating graft is an option.

Prognosis

• Fair. Surgical treatment has a low success rate.

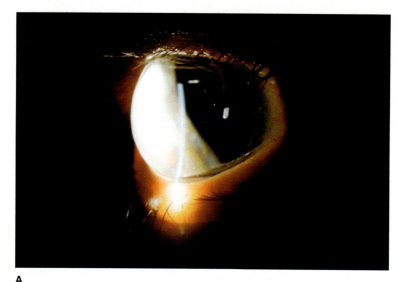

A

B

Figure 4-3 Keratoglobus **A.** *A thin, bulging cornea is evident in this eye with keratoglobus.* **B.** *A slit-lamp view of the eye shown in Figure 4-3A demonstrates that the thinnest portion of the cornea is in the periphery in this eye with keratoglobus.*

Chapter 5

CORNEAL DYSTROPHIES

ANTERIOR CORNEAL DYSTROPHIES

ANTERIOR BASEMENT MEMBRANE DYSTROPHY (MAP-DOT-FINGERPRINT DYSTROPHY, COGAN'S MICROCYSTIC DYSTROPHY)

Anterior basement (ABM) dystrophy is a common epithelial dystrophy that can cause painful recurrent corneal erosions and/or decreased vision.

Etiology and Pathology

- ABM dystrophy is due to an abnormality of production of epithelial basement membrane that extends into the epithelium, leading to multiple basement membranes in the corneal epithelium. Trapped epithelial cells can form "Cogan's microcysts."

Symptoms

- Most commonly asymptomatic
- Recurrent erosion syndrome: may have unilateral or bilateral recurrent episodes of pain in the middle of the night or upon opening the eyes after sleep. Can occur after trauma with a sharp object such as a fingernail, tree branch, or paper edge.
- May note painless distortion of vision when the central cornea is involved.

Signs

- Slit-lamp examination shows maplike lines, dots (microcysts), and/or fingerprintlike epithelial lesions, which may occur singly or in various combinations. These findings are best seen with retroillumination and with a broad slit beam from the side. There may be "negative staining" from slightly elevated areas of epithelium seen with fluorescein dye (Figures 5-1A,B,C,D).
- Eyes with recurrent erosions may have minimal clinical findings, localized areas of loose epithelium, or a frank epithelial defect.

Differential Diagnosis

- Other anterior corneal dystrophies, such as Meesmann's dystrophy and Reis-Bücklers' dystrophy

Treatment

- If vision is decreased due to central involvement, the irregular epithelium can be debrided.
- Painful erosions can be treated with lubrication, hypertonic drops and ointment (sodium chloride 5%), pressure patching, debridement, bandage soft contact lens, anterior stromal micropuncture, diamond burr polishing of Bowman's membrane, or excimer laser phototherapeutic keratectomy (PTK).

Prognosis

- Very good with appropriate treatment, although some patients have recalcitrant recurrent erosions

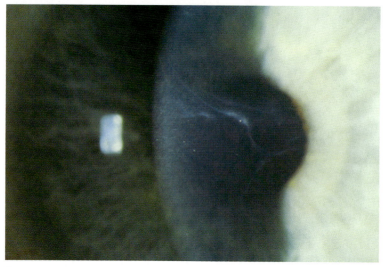

A

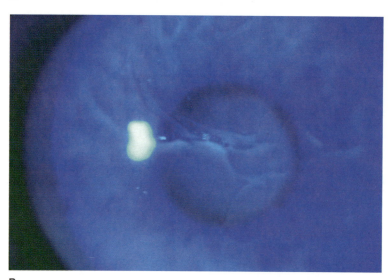

B

Figure 5-1   Anterior basement membrane dystrophy   *A. Maplike changes due to anterior basement membrane dystrophy. Note the "mare's tail" pattern of multiple epithelial layers.*
B. Fluorescein stain and the cobalt blue light view of the cornea in **Figure 5-1A**. *Significant "negative staining" is evident due to areas of elevated epithelium. These elevated areas can cause foreign body sensation and/or decreased vision. (Continued.)*

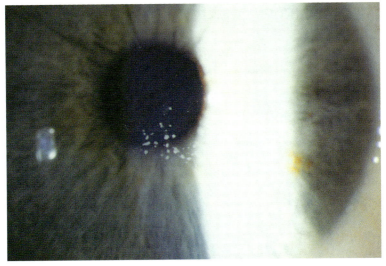

C

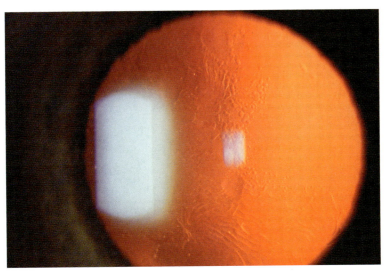

D

Figure 5-1 (cont.)   Anterior basement membrane dystrophy   C. *Dot changes of ABM dystrophy. These creamy white Cogan's microcysts are tiny pockets of surface epithelial cells trapped beneath an abnormal epithelial basement membrane.* **D.** *Fingerprintlike changes of ABM dystrophy in retroillumination. These parallel lines and bleblike changes are due to irregularities in the epithelial basement membrane. They can cause irregular astigmatism and decreased vision.*

MEESMANN'S DYSTROPHY (HEREDITARY JUVENILE EPITHELIAL DYSTROPHY)

Meesmann's dystrophy is a rare bilateral epithelial disorder that can cause ocular irritation and photophobia.

Etiology and Pathology

- Meesmann's dystrophy is an autosomal dominant condition in which hundreds of tiny vesicles containing periodic acid-Schiff (PAS)-positive "peculiar substance" develop in the epithelium.

Symptoms

- Patients are usually asymptomatic, but may note irritation, glare, and photophobia. Mild pain may develop in adulthood due to recurrent corneal erosions.

Signs

- Retroillumination demonstrates myriad tiny, translucent, epithelial cysts that extend to the limbus and are most numerous in the interpalpebral region. The lesions appear gray or clear under direct illumination (Figures 5-2A,B).

Treatment

- Most patients require no treatment. Consider lubrication and sunglasses for mild symptoms. Rarely, a bandage soft contact lens can be used or a superficial keratectomy can be performed for severe symptoms, but the dystrophy will recur.

Prognosis

- Good, although rare patients will have chronic symptoms

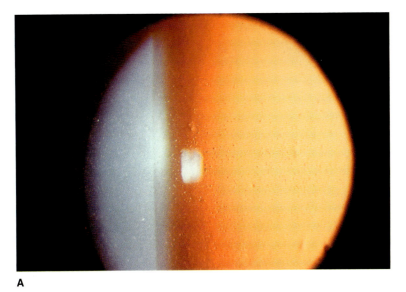

A

B

Figure 5-2 Meesmann's dystrophy A. *Multiple tiny, translucent, epithelial cysts are apparent in retroillumination. They tend to be more prominent in the interpalpebral zone.* B. *On direct illumination, the microcysts are gray in color but are difficult to see. On illumination off the iris, at the 3 o'clock edge of the pupil, myriad microcysts are visible.*

REIS-BÜCKLERS' DYSTROPHY

Reis-Bücklers' dystrophy is an uncommon, bilateral, symmetric dystrophy of Bowman's membrane that causes pain and decreased vision early in life.

Etiology

- Reis-Bücklers' dystrophy is an autosomal dominant (Big h3 gene, chromosome 5q31) disorder causing damage and scarring to Bowman's membrane and the anterior stroma.

Symptoms

- Severe recurrent corneal erosions from a young age, even soon after birth.
- Progression of the condition leads to reduced visual acuity that occurs in the second to third decades of life, although in severe cases it can occur in the first decade.

Signs

- Honeycomb appearance due to reticular, ring-shaped, subepithelial opacities that are most dense centrally but may involve the entire cornea. With time, they can progress deeper into the stroma (Figures 5-3A,B).

Differential Diagnosis

- Other anterior or stromal dystrophies (e.g., anterior basement membrane dystrophy, granular dystrophy, macular dystrophy)

Treatment

- Mild cases: lubrication.
- More severe cases: bandage soft contact lenses, superficial keratectomy, excimer laser PTK, lamellar keratoplasty, or penetrating keratoplasty may be necessary.

Prognosis

- Excimer laser PTK can be quite successful in improving vision and decreasing painful episodes in many cases. Keratoplasty may be required in advanced cases. Recurrence in the donor graft is common after corneal transplant and also after PTK (Figure 5-3C). PTK can often be repeated or performed for recurrence after keratoplasty.

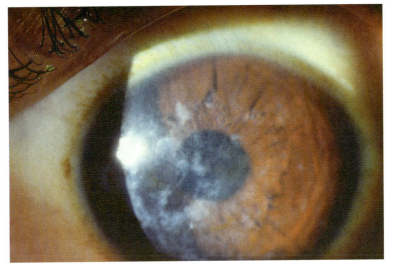

A

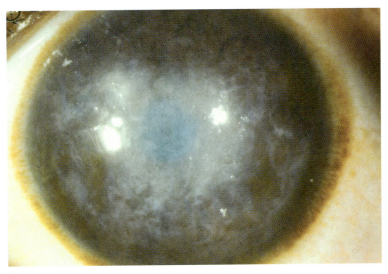

B

Figure 5-3 Reis-Bücklers' dystrophy A. *This eye has moderate changes of Reis-Bücklers' dystrophy. It primarily involves the central cornea, but the opacity approaches the limbus inferiorly.* B. *This eye with advanced Reis-Bücklers' dystrophy has diffuse, reticular, limbus-to-limbus subepithelial and anterior stromal opacity. There are few if any clear spaces. (Continued.)*

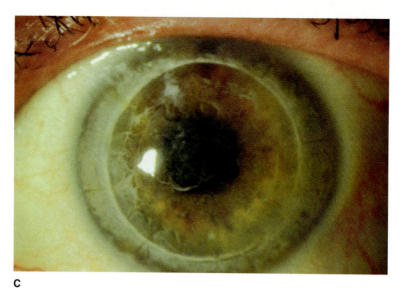

C

Figure 5-3 (cont.)   Reis-Bücklers' dystrophy   C. *This eye has recurrent Reis-Bücklers'
dystrophy several years after penetrating keratoplasty. Note the honeycomb opacity centrally and
involvement of the entire corneal periphery.*

STROMAL CORNEAL DYSTROPHIES

GRANULAR DYSTROPHY

Granular dystrophy is an uncommon disorder that can cause decreased vision and recurrent painful erosions in young adults.

Etiology and Pathology

- Granular dystrophy is an autosomal dominant (Big h3 gene, chromosome 5q31) disorder which becomes manifest during the first or second decade of life.

Histopathology Hyaline deposits stain bright red with Masson trichrome.

Symptoms

- Painful recurrent erosions are uncommon, but may occur before the vision is significantly affected.
- Decreased vision occurs in young adulthood and middle age, when the corneal opacities become confluent.

Signs

- Small, discrete, white granules ("crushed breadcrumbs") within the central anterior stroma, separated by clear intervening spaces. With time, the lesions extend deeper within the stroma and become larger and more numerous. With more time, superficial lesions become confluent over the pupillary axis, severely affecting vision. The periphery is spared (Figures 5-4A,B,C,D,E,F).

Differential Diagnosis

- Other anterior or stromal dystrophies (e.g., Reis-Bücklers' dystrophy, macular dystrophy)

Treatment

Mild cases: lubrication

More severe cases: bandage soft contact lenses, superficial keratectomy, excimer laser PTK, lamellar keratoplasty, or penetrating keratoplasty may be necessary

Prognosis

- Excimer laser PTK can be quite successful in improving vision and decreasing painful episodes in many cases. Keratoplasty may be required in advanced cases. Recurrence in the donor graft is common after corneal transplantation and also after PTK, although it takes longer than after surgery for Reis-Bücklers' dystrophy. PTK can often be repeated or performed for recurrence after keratoplasty.

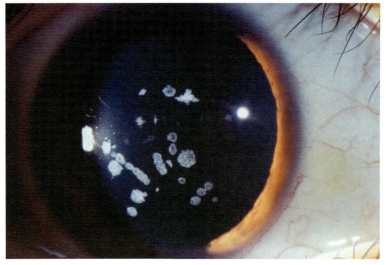

A

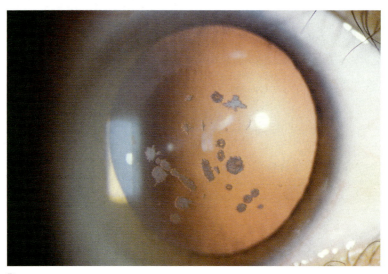

B

Figure 5-4 Granular dystrophy *A. This eye with mild granular dystrophy has minimal opacity and still retains excellent vision. There are numerous discrete white, "crushed breadcrumb" opacities centrally with clear intervening spaces.* **B.** *This is the same eye as in Figure 5-4A seen in retroillumination off the retina; the granules are highlighted. (Continued.)*

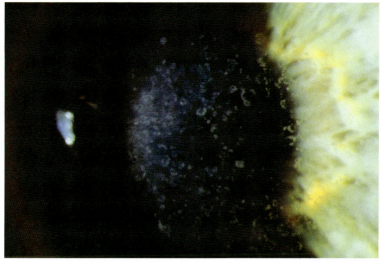

C

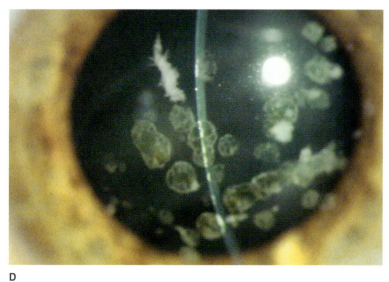

D

Figure 5-4 (cont.) **Granular dystrophy** C. *This eye with granular dystrophy has relatively confluent opacities although the granules are small and not very dense.* **D.** *This slit-lamp view demonstrates some of the granular opacities to be rather superficial. (Continued.)*

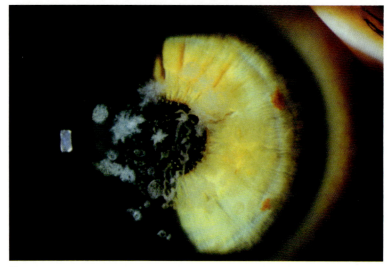

E

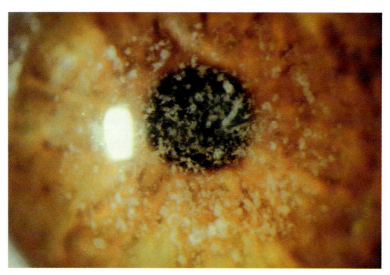

F

Figure 5-4 (cont.) Granular dystrophy *E. This eye has a combination of the flat "crushed breadcrumb" opacities and the more three-dimensional dense white stellate opacities. The intervening spaces are still relatively clear. F. The larger, denser, deeper granules are hidden by almost confluent, very anterior stromal opacities. The vision is poor. Fortunately, the confluent anterior opacities are often treatable with excimer laser PTK.*

LATTICE DYSTROPHY

Lattice dystrophy is an uncommon disorder that typically causes recurrent painful erosions in young adults and decreased vision later in life.

Etiology and Pathology

Lattice dystrophy can be subdivided into three types:

Type I Autosomal dominant inheritance (Big h3 gene, chromosome 5q31). Fine, branching, refractile lines within the anterior or midstroma, sparing the corneal periphery. By far the most common form.

Type II (Meretoja's Syndrome) Associated with systemic amyloidosis and has autosomal dominant inheritance. Lattice lines are thicker but less numerous than in type I; the lines begin peripherally and progress centrally. Visual acuity is usually good, with minimal recurrent erosions.

Type III Autosomal recessive inheritance. Lattice lines are coarser than in type I and go from limbus to limbus. No recurrent erosions.

Histopathology Amyloid deposits, stain pinkish red with Congo red dye, metachromatic with crystal violet stain, and demonstrate apple-green birefringence when viewed with polarized light.

Symptoms

- Painful recurrent corneal erosions are common and can occur in childhood or early adulthood. Vision typically declines after early adulthood.

Signs

- Central, branching, refractile lines (seen well with retroillumination), subepithelial white dots, and diffuse anterior stromal haze can be seen early in the disease. Later, significant subepithelial fibrosis and scarring can occur (Figures 5-5A,B,C,D).

Differential Diagnosis

- Polymorphic amyloid degeneration (PAD): a condition of older patients with no painful erosions, no decreased vision, and no family history of cornea problems. Few or many refractile amyloid dots or lines are seen in the stroma, typically centrally.

Treatment

- Mild cases: lubrication

- More severe cases: bandage soft contact lenses, superficial keratectomy, excimer laser PTK, lamellar keratoplasty, or penetrating keratoplasty may be necessary

Prognosis

- Excimer laser PTK can be successful in improving vision and decreasing painful episodes in certain cases. Keratoplasty may be required in others. Recurrence in the donor graft is common after corneal transplant and also after PTK, although it takes longer than after surgery for Reis-Bücklers' dystrophy. PTK can often be repeated or performed for recurrence after keratoplasty.

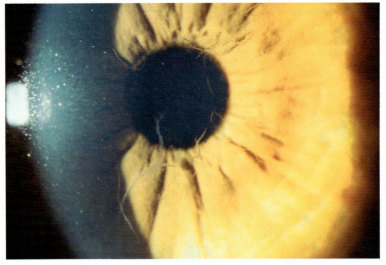

A

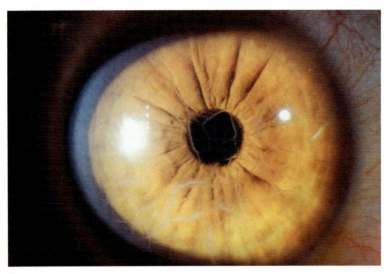

B

Figure 5-5 Lattice dystrophy A. *This eye has mild type I lattice dystrophy. Note the fine, branching lines that appear gray-white on direct illumination and refractile on retroillumination off the iris.* **B.** *This eye with type I lattice dystrophy has moderately advanced disease. There are multiple, relatively thick lattice lines centrally and in the midperiphery. (Continued.)*

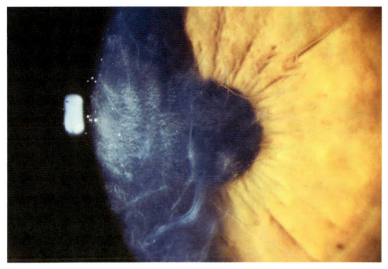

C

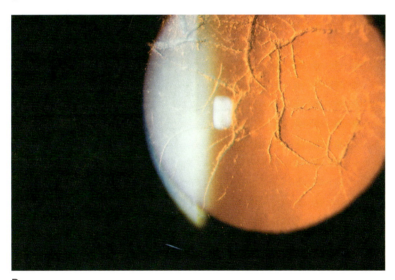

D

Figure 5-5 (cont.)   Lattice dystrophy   C. *This eye with type I lattice dystrophy has central anterior stromal haze due to numerous previous episodes of recurrent erosions. There is subepithelial fibrosis centrally. Often, this scarring leads to diminished recurrent erosions but greatly impedes vision. Refractile lattice lines are still visible.* **D.** *Retroillumination off the retina highlights the refractile amyloid deposits in lattice dystrophy.*

MACULAR DYSTROPHY

Macular dystrophy is a rare disorder that typically causes glare and decreased vision in young adult life.

Etiology and Pathology

Macular dystrophy is an autosomal recessive disorder mapped to chromosome 16q22. It can be subdivided into two types through blood testing:

Type I   Presents in childhood and is more common and lacks keratan sulfate in the cornea.

Type II   Presents in the second decade, and keratan sulfate is present in the cornea.

Histopathology   Acid mucopolysaccharide (glycosaminoglycan) deposits which stain with colloidal iron and Alcian blue stains.

Symptoms

- Glare and decreased vision in young adults.
- May have painful recurrent erosion symptoms.

Signs

- Central, gray-white, ill-defined but relatively focal opacities with diffuse cloudiness of the intervening stroma. The cornea is usually thinner than normal. The lesions extend from limbus to limbus and eventually involve the entire stromal thickness. The central lesions are superficial while the peripheral lesions are deep (Figures 5-6A,B,C).

Differential Diagnosis

- Other anterior or stromal dystrophies (e.g., Reis-Bücklers' dystrophy, granular dystrophy)

Treatment

- Vision is usually affected by the third decade and requires a corneal transplant. Excimer laser PTK may be helpful on rare occasion.

Prognosis

- Good with corneal transplantation. Recurrence after keratoplasty is uncommon and occurs late.

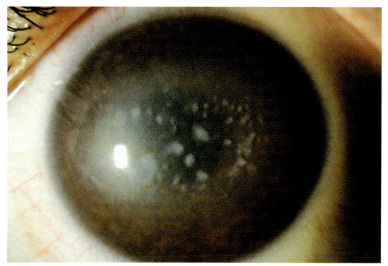

A

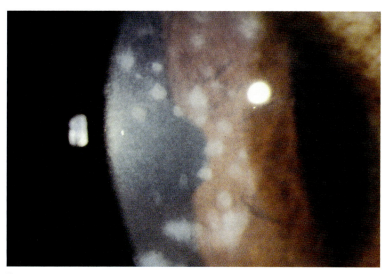

B

Figure 5-6   Macular dystrophy   A. *This eye with macular dystrophy has central opacities of various shapes and sizes. While faint, these opacities are also present in the corneal periphery. The entire central cornea is involved with a confluent stromal opacity, so there are no clear zones between the dense macules.* **B.** *In this eye the central and peripheral opacities are very apparent. The entire cornea is involved with a diffuse full thickness haze. (Continued.)*

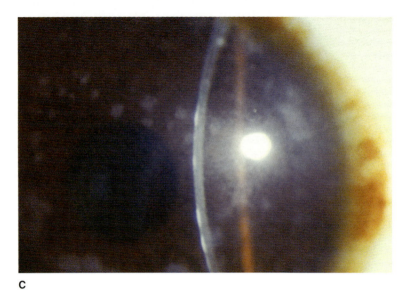

C

Figure 5-6 (cont.)   Macular dystrophy   C. *Slit-lamp view demonstrates that the central opacities are in the anterior stroma and the peripheral opacities are in the posterior stroma. This distribution is a classic finding in macular dystrophy. The full-thickness corneal haze is also visible.*

AVELLINO DYSTROPHY

Avellino dystrophy is a rare variant of granular dystrophy with significant amyloid deposition similar to lattice dystrophy. It causes symptoms similar to those of granular dystrophy.

Etiology and Pathology

- Avellino dystrophy is an autosomal dominant (Big h3 gene, chromosome 5q31) disorder that becomes manifest during the first few decades of life.

Histopathology   Consists of both hyaline and amyloid deposits.

Symptoms

- Painful recurrent erosions are more common than in granular dystrophy.
- Decreased vision occurs in middle age, when the central corneal opacities become confluent.

Signs

- Anterior stromal "crushed breadcrumb" opacities suggestive of granular dystrophy, associated with deeper stromal refractile lines similar to those found in lattice dystrophy (Figures 5-7A,B)

Differential Diagnosis

- Other anterior or stromal dystrophies (e.g., Reis-Bücklers' dystrophy, granular dystrophy, lattice dystrophy, macular dystrophy)

Treatment

- Mild cases: lubrication
- More severe cases: bandage soft contact lenses, superficial keratectomy, excimer laser PTK, lamellar keratoplasty, or penetrating keratoplasty may be necessary.

Prognosis

- Excimer laser PTK can be quite successful in improving vision and decreasing painful episodes in many cases. Keratoplasty may be required in advanced cases. Recurrence in the donor graft is common after corneal transplant and also after PTK, although it takes longer than after surgery for Reis-Bücklers' dystrophy. PTK can often be repeated or performed for recurrence after keratoplasty.

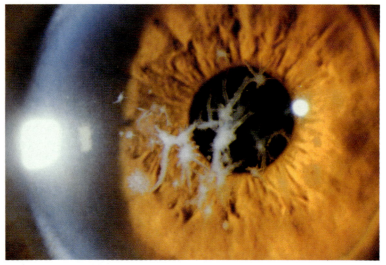

A

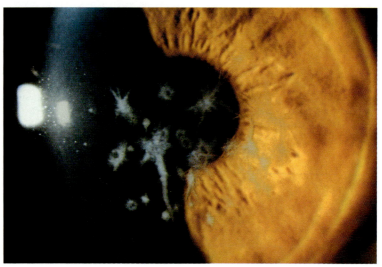

B

Figure 5-7   Avellino dystrophy   A. *This right eye demonstrates characteristics of both granular and lattice dystrophy. There are several "crushed breadcrumb" opacities along with the refractile lines of lattice dystrophy.* **B.** *The left eye of the patient shown in* **Figure 5-7A** *has similar features to those of the right eye.*

SCHNYDER'S CRYSTALLINE DYSTROPHY

Schnyder's crystalline dystrophy is a condition related to cholesterol deposition in the cornea. There are few ocular symptoms until late in life, although the deposits may be seen early.

Etiology

- This is an uncommon, autosomal dominant condition associated with hypercholesterolemia and hypertriglyceridemia. Mapped to chromosome 1.
- It can be associated with systemic hyperlipidemia or hypercholesterolemia. Also associated with genu valgum and xanthelasma.

Symptoms

- Glare symptoms in adulthood. In severe cases, patients can develop decreased vision.

Signs

- Fine ring of yellowish-white crystalline cholesterol deposits mainly involving the central anterior stroma (Figures 5-8A,B).
- Often associated with a prominent arcus lipoides.
- A full-thickness central stromal haze develops in later stages (Figure 5-8C).

Differential Diagnosis

- Other causes of corneal crystals (e.g., infectious crystalline keratopathy, cystinosis, gout, multiple myeloma, monoclonal gammopathies)

Treatment

- Check fasting cholesterol and triglyceride levels.
- Excimer laser PTK or corneal transplantation is rarely needed late in life in eyes with severe corneal opacity.

Prognosis

- Vision is usually good and corneal transplant is usually not necessary. PTK can be used to remove the superficial crystals in patients with severe glare. Recurrence after PTK or keratoplasty is rare.

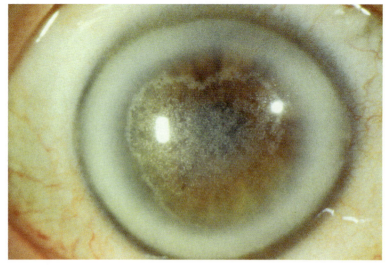

A

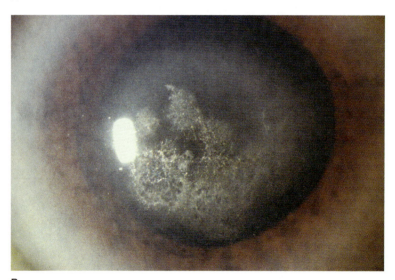

B

Figure 5-8   Schnyder's crystalline dystrophy   A. *The three classic characteristics of Schnyder's crystalline dystrophy are evident in this eye. The central, superficial crystalline opacities, full-thickness stromal haze, and dense peripheral arcus lipoides are all apparent. The central crystals can have a more dense annular pattern as in this eye.* **B.** *In this high-magnification view, the superficial crystals and underlying stromal haze are visible. The edge of the arcus lipoides can also be seen. (Continued.)*

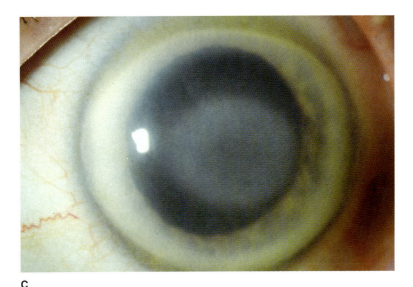

C

Figure 5-8 (cont.) **Schnyder's crystalline dystrophy** **C.** *This patient, with a family history of Schnyder's crystalline dystrophy, had the noncrystalline form. The central full-thickness opacity and arcus lipoides are present.*

POSTERIOR CORNEAL DYSTROPHIES

ENDOTHELIAL DYSTROPHY AND FUCHS' DYSTROPHY

Endothelial dystrophy and Fuchs' dystrophy represent a continuum of disease involving abnormalities in Descemet's membrane that affect the endothelial cells. Before stromal edema occurs, the condition is termed endothelial dystrophy; after stromal edema develops, it is termed Fuchs' dystrophy.

Etiology, Epidemiology, and Pathology

- Endothelial dystrophy is a common condition that may proceed to Fuchs' dystrophy over a period of years.
- Fuchs' dystrophy occurs after the fifth or sixth decade, more commonly in women.
- Inheritance is typically autosomal dominant but can be recessive.

Histopathology   Tiny, central excrescences of a thickened Descemet's membrane known as cornea guttata; pigment on the endothelium.

Specular Microscopy   Variable endothelial size and shape, numerous dark areas, reduced number of endothelial cells.

Symptoms

- Asymptomatic in endothelial dystrophy and early stages of Fuchs' dystrophy.
- Mild visual loss develops later as posterior stromal edema increases. When epithelial edema develops, there is often a significant decrease in vision. Patients often have worse vision upon awakening in the morning, which improves over several hours.
- As epithelial edema worsens, bullae, which can rupture, can cause severe pain.

Signs

- Tiny, central excrescences of Descemet's membrane known as cornea guttata are seen. The confluence of lesions gives rise to a "beaten-metal" appearance (Figures 5-9A,B).

- A variable amount of pigment on the endothelium and a gray, thickened appearance of Descemet's membrane (Figure 5-9C).
- Stromal edema develops, giving rise to a thickened cornea (Fuchs' dystrophy).
- Epithelial edema and bullae (bullous keratopathy) form, which may rupture causing irritation and pain. Years of bullae formation can cause scarring and fibrosis, with fewer painful symptoms, but poorer vision (Figure 5-9D).
- Increased incidence of hyperopia, narrow angles, and glaucoma.

Differential Diagnosis

- Aphakic and pseudophakic bullous keratopathy: after cataract surgery
- Posterior polymorphous dystrophy: linear, band-like, vesicular, or grouped configurations with irregular edges at the level of Descemet's membrane

Treatment

- Treatment in early stages includes hypertonic saline, lubrication, and lowering intraocular pressure. When mild epithelial edema is present, blowing warm air from a hair dryer held at arm's length over the eyes for 5 to 10 minutes each morning can improve some patients' vision earlier in the day. When vision is significantly impaired, penetrating keratoplasty (or more recently, posterior lamellar keratoplasty) is indicated.

Prognosis

- Endothelial dystrophy uncommonly progresses to Fuchs' dystrophy. Cataract surgery may precipitate development of permanent corneal edema in eyes with endothelial dystrophy. Mild to moderate Fuchs' dystrophy can often be managed successfully without surgery, but if a corneal transplant is required, the success rate is very good.

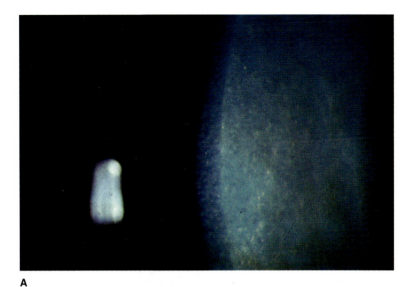

A

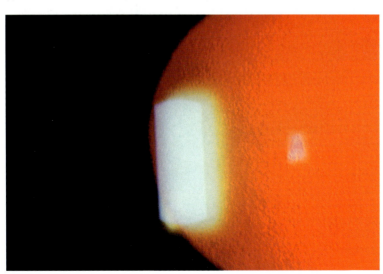

B

Figure 5-9   Fuchs' dystrophy   A. *Using high magnification, a thickened Descemet's membrane with a corrugated pattern to the endothelial cell layer is apparent.* **B.** *Using retroillumination off the retina, the "beaten-metal" pattern of cornea guttata can easily be appreciated. (Continued.)*

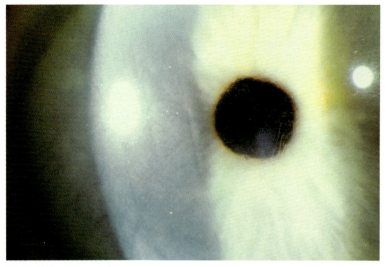

C

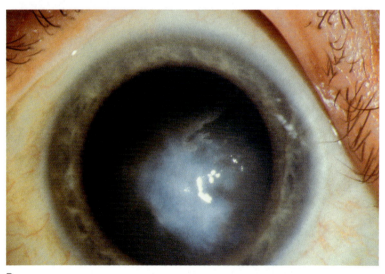

D

Figure 5-9 (cont.)   Fuchs' dystrophy   C. *This eye with mild Fuchs' dystrophy has mild stromal edema with some Descemet's folds. There are some secondary epithelial basement membrane changes at the 5 o'clock edge of the pupil. Brown pigment on the endothelium can be seen centrally.* **D.** *This eye with advanced Fuchs' dystrophy has developed stromal edema involving most of the central cornea. A large area of elevated subepithelial fibrosis is present in the central area of the edema.*

POSTERIOR POLYMORPHOUS DYSTROPHY

Posterior polymorphous dystrophy is an uncommon condition characterized by various abnormalities of Descemet's membrane and the endothelium.

Etiology and Pathology

- This is an uncommon, autosomal dominant, markedly variable condition affecting Descemet's membrane and endothelium. The signs and symptoms can be very variable even within a family.

Histopathology Endothelial cells look like epithelial cells in that they have microvilli and stain positive for keratin.

Symptoms

- Onset of symptoms may occur at birth, but many patients are asymptomatic.
- The main symptom is decreased vision due to corneal edema. Pain can occur if corneal bullae develop.

Signs

- Linear, bandlike, vesicular, or grouped configurations with irregular, often scalloped edges at the level of Descemet's membrane. The lesions are frequently asymmetric. There may be corneal edema in advanced cases (Figures 5-10A,B,C).
- Of those affected, 15% have glaucoma. May be associated with iridocorneal adhesions and corectopia.
- May be associated with Alport's syndrome (hereditary nephritis and sensorineural hearing loss).

Differential Diagnosis

- Iridocorneal endothelial syndrome: unilateral and nonhereditary

Treatment

- Most patients require no treatment. Patients need to be monitored for glaucoma.
- If corneal edema develops, it can be treated similarly to Fuchs' dystrophy. When vision is significantly impaired, penetrating keratoplasty (or more recently, posterior lamellar keratoplasty) is indicated.

Prognosis

- Very good for retaining good vision. When significant iris changes are present, the chances of glaucoma increase. Posterior polymorphous dystrophy rarely requires corneal transplantation, but if a corneal transplant is required, the success rate is good.

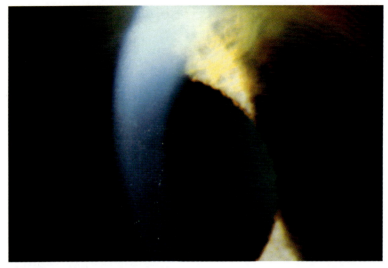

A

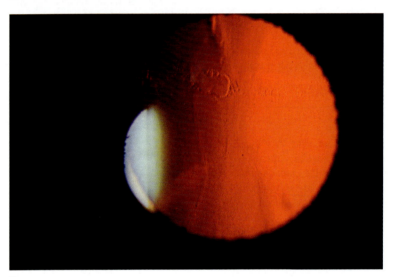

B

Figure 5-10 Posterior polymorphous dystrophy **A.** *On direct illumination, a scalloped band in the endothelium is visible just superior to the visual axis.* **B.** *On retroillumination of the retina, the scalloped band seen in Figure 5-10A is more apparent. (Continued.)*

CHAPTER 5. CORNEAL DYSTROPHIES

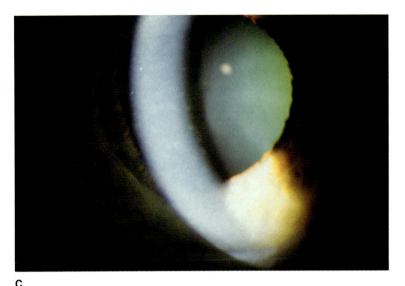

C

Figure 5-10 (cont.)   Posterior polymorphous dystrophy   C. *Multiple small gray areas are evident on the endothelial surface in this eye with posterior polymorphous dystrophy.*

CONGENITAL HEREDITARY ENDOTHELIAL DYSTROPHY (CHED)

Congenital hereditary endothelial dystrophy is an extremely rare condition involving corneal edema at birth or shortly thereafter.

Etiology and Pathology

- Autosomal recessive and autosomal dominant forms have been described.

Histopathology Abnormal or absent endothelial cells.

Symptoms

Autosomal Recessive Form Presents at birth, is nonprogressive, nystagmus is present, and there is no pain

Autosomal Dominant Form Presents in the first 1 to 2 years of life, is progressive, with no nystagmus, but pain and photophobia are common

Signs

- Bilateral, limbus-to-limbus corneal stromal edema with a blue-gray ground glass appearance (Figure 5-11)
- Corneal thickness can be 2 to 3 times normal
- No increase in corneal diameter or elevated intraocular pressure

Differential Diagnosis

- Congenital glaucoma: enlarged corneal diameter, elevated intraocular pressure
- Birth trauma: unilateral, parallel oblique breaks in Descemet's membrane

Treatment

- Depends on degree of corneal edema. Penetrating keratoplasty may be indicated if corneal edema is severe.

Prognosis

- Fair, due to the difficulty of performing corneal transplantation in children.

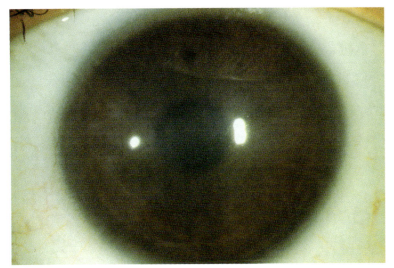

Figure 5-11   Congenital hereditary endothelial dystrophy   *Diffuse limbus-to-limbus corneal edema with a blue-gray ground glass appearance is present in this eye with congenital hereditary endothelial dystrophy.*

Chapter 6

CORNEAL DEGENERATIONS AND DEPOSITS

INVOLUTIONAL CHANGES

CORNEAL ARCUS

- Corneal arcus is a very common, bilateral condition that may be either age-related (arcus senilis) or associated with hyperlipidemia in younger individuals (arcus lipoides).
- Lipid deposits begin inferiorly, then superiorly, and later extend circumferentially to form a white perilimbal band about 1 mm in diameter with a sharp outline peripherally and a more diffuse boundary centrally. A clear zone of cornea separates it from the limbus (Figure 6-1A).
- May be accompanied by mild, nonprogressive thinning of the clear zone of cornea (furrow degeneration).
- Check for hyperlipidemia in patients under age 40 years. If unilateral, check for carotid disease on the uninvolved side.
- Patients are asymptomatic and ocular treatment is not necessary.

WHITE LIMBAL GIRDLE OF VOGT

- White limbal girdle of Vogt is a very common, bilateral, innocuous, age-related condition characterized by chalky-white, crescentic deposits (elastotic degeneration) along the nasal and temporal perilimbal cornea. It may or may not be separated from the limbus by a clear zone (Figure 6-1B).
- Patients are asymptomatic and ocular treatment is not necessary.

CROCODILE SHAGREEN

- Crocodile shagreen is characterized by grayish-white, polygonal stromal opacities separated by relatively clear spaces. The lesions usually involve the anterior stroma (anterior crocodile shagreen), but they may also be found more posteriorly (posterior crocodile shagreen) (Figure 6-1C).
- Patients are asymptomatic and ocular treatment is not necessary.

CORNEA FARINATA

- Cornea farinata is a relatively common condition characterized by bilateral, innocuous, minute, "flour-dust" lipofuscinlike deposits in the deep stroma near Descemet's membrane. It is most prominent centrally.
- These opacities are best seen with retroillumination off the iris (Figure 6-1D).
- Patients are asymptomatic and ocular treatment is not necessary.

POLYMORPHIC AMYLOID DEGENERATION

- Polymorphic amyloid degeneration is a fairly common, bilateral, innocuous, degenerative condition usually seen after the age of 50 years.
- It is characterized by polymorphic, refractile, punctate, comma-shaped and filamentous amyloid deposits throughout the stroma, but are generally most prominent centrally and posteriorly. These deposits are best seen with retroillumination off the retina (Figures 6-1E,F).
- It is not associated with any systemic disorder.
- Differential diagnosis: cornea farinata and lattice dystrophy.
- Patients are asymptomatic and ocular treatment is not necessary.

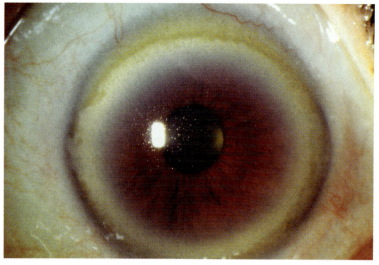

A

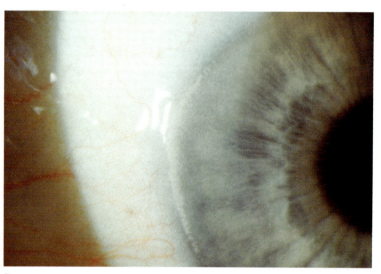

B

Figure 6-1 Corneal arcus A. *A circular yellow-white lipid deposition is present adjacent to the limbus for 360 degrees. Note the clear zone between the arcus and the limbus.* **Limbal girdle of Vogt** B. *A crescentic, relatively dense white opacity is seen at the limbus at the 9 o'clock position. There is a small clear zone between the limbal girdle and the limbus. (Continued.)*

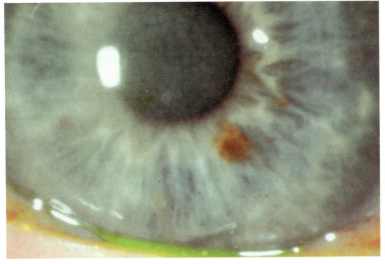

C

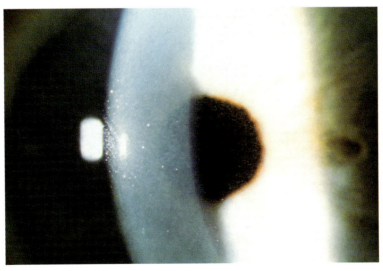

D

Figure 6-1 (cont.) Crocodile shagreen C. *Gray-white polygonal stromal opacities are evident in this corneal transplant. They may be located in the anterior or the posterior stroma.*
Cornea farinata D. *Tiny, "flour-dust" deposits are seen at the pupillary margin. These pinpoint opacities are located in the deep stroma. They do not affect vision. (Continued.)*

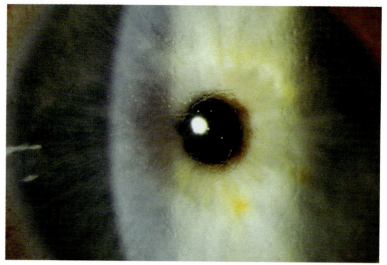

E

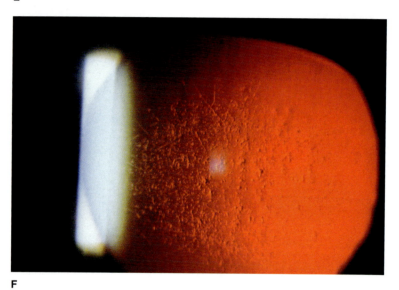

F

Figure 6-1 (cont.) Polymorphic amyloid degeneration *E. Amyloid deposits in various shapes, including dots, commas, and lines, are seen in the corneal stroma. This condition is a degeneration, not a dystrophy. It is similar to lattice dystrophy in that they both involve amyloid deposition; however, lattice dystrophy is an inherited condition that is typically associated with recurrent erosions and decreased vision in young adulthood. F. This eye with polymorphic amyloid degeneration has dense central amyloid deposits readily seen in retroillumination off the retina.*

CORNEAL DEPOSITS—NONPIGMENTED

BAND KERATOPATHY

Band keratopathy is a common condition characterized by calcium deposits in the subepithelial space, Bowman's layer, and anterior stroma.

Etiology

Ocular
- Chronic ocular inflammation (e.g., iridocyclitis, juvenile rheumatoid arthritis, corneal edema, interstitial keratitis, phthisis bulbi)
- Silicone oil in the anterior chamber

Metabolic
- Hypercalcemia or hyperphosphatemia
- Gout
- Chronic renal failure

Hereditary Familial

Other
- Chronic exposure to toxic vapors (e.g., mercury)
- Idiopathic (age-related)

Symptoms

- Often asymptomatic. If central, vision may be affected. Ocular irritation can develop if thick calcium plaques flake off and cause an epithelial defect.

Signs

- Peripheral, interpalpebral plaque of calcium deposit separated from the limbus by a thin line of clear cornea (Figures 6-2A,B,C).
- The plaque typically begins at the nasal and temporal cornea and extends centrally.
- It often contains small holes and clefts giving it a swiss-cheese appearance.
- Advanced lesions may become plaquelike, nodular, and elevated.

Treatment

- Mild cases may be observed or treated with lubricants (e.g., artificial tear drops or ointments).
- Severe cases (with visual, painful, or cosmetic indications) can be treated with chelation using disodium ethylenediamine tetraacetic acid 3% or superficial keratectomy.

Prognosis

Excellent for the ocular calcium deposits. The band keratopathy can recur, especially if the underlying condition persists. Calcium chelation can be repeated if necessary. Epithelial healing problems may occur. Vision is often limited from other ocular pathology.

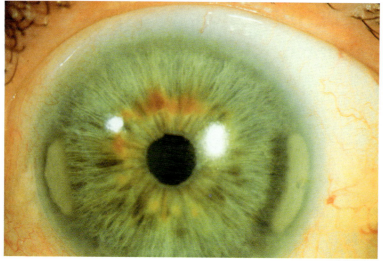

A

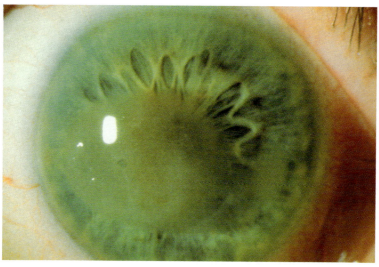

B

Figure 6-2 Band keratopathy **A.** *A thin layer of calcium deposition can be seen adjacent to the limbus nasally and temporally. Note the thin line of clear cornea between the band keratopathy and the limbus.* **B.** *This eye had central calcium deposition obscuring the view of the iris and pupil. (Continued.)*

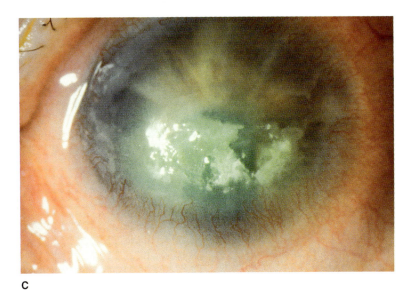

C

Figure 6-2 (cont.) Band keratopathy   C. *This eye with chronic corneal edema has a dense central plaque of calcium deposition. Some of the plaque spontaneously flaked off centrally.*

SALZMANN'S NODULAR DEGENERATION

Salzmann's nodular degeneration is an uncommon, usually unilateral condition characterized by smooth gray-white elevated lesions of the cornea.

Etiology

- It is typically found in eyes with a history of chronic keratopathy, such as interstitial keratitis, vernal keratoconjunctivitis, keratoconjunctivitis sicca, phlyctenulosis, and trachoma, but may appear in otherwise normal eyes.

Symptoms

- Often asymptomatic. May affect vision if it becomes central; rarely causes a foreign body sensation if it becomes very elevated.

Signs

- Single or multiple, discrete, white or gray-white, smooth, elevated nodules anywhere on the surface of the cornea (Figure 6-3).
- Longstanding nodules may have iron pigment deposition at the base of the nodule.

Differential Diagnosis

- Spheroidal degeneration: small, globular, yellow-brown granules are found in the superficial corneal stroma

Treatment

- Mild cases are observed or treated with lubrication. If causing symptoms, the nodules may be treated with superficial keratectomy or excimer laser phototherapeutic keratectomy (PTK). Rarely, if severe it may require a lamellar keratoplasty.

Prognosis

- Very good to excellent. Can recur after surgical excision.

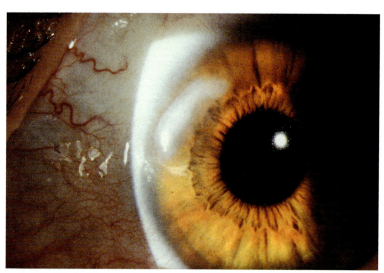

Figure 6-3   Salzmann's nodular degeneration   *A gray-white elevated lesion is seen in the peripheral cornea from the 9 to 11 o'clock positions. These lesions may be single or multiple and peripheral or central. If causing symptoms, they can usually be treated with a superficial keratectomy or less commonly with excimer laser PTK.*

OTHER CORNEAL DEGENERATIONS

SPHEROIDAL DEGENERATION

(Labrador's Keratopathy, Actinic Keratopathy, Climatic Droplet Keratopathy, Corneal Elastosis, Bietti's Nodular Dystrophy)

- Spheroidal degeneration is a rare, bilateral condition that typically affects people who work outdoors.
- Interpalpebral, small, globular, yellow-brown granules are found in the superficial corneal stroma (Figure 6-4A).
- The lesions often begin peripherally and progress centrally. Advanced lesions can become nodular and elevated.
- Vision becomes affected when lesions are central. Patients can develop a foreign body sensation from elevated nodules.
- When vision becomes impaired, treatment is with superficial keratectomy, phototherapeutic keratectomy, or lamellar or penetrating keratoplasty. Lesions may recur.

LIPID KERATOPATHY

- This is a relatively common unilateral condition most frequently associated with previous herpes zoster or herpes simplex keratitis.
- Unilateral, focal, white or yellowish deposits with feathery edges. Secondary lesions are associated with vascularization, whereas primary lesions are avascular. May appear crystalline. Rarely, the lipid may involve the entire cornea (Figures 6-4B,C).
- Vision can be affected by central lipid deposition.
- Treatment is with topical corticosteroids to decrease inflammation and vascularization. Laser ablation of vessels can be attempted but they typically reopen. Advanced cases may require corneal transplant.

COATS' WHITE RING

- Small, oval, white ring, 1 mm or less in diameter, usually located in the inferior cornea at the level of Bowman's layer with an intact overlying epithelium (Figure 6-4D).
- Represents old metallic foreign body injury.
- Patients are asymptomatic and ocular treatment is not necessary.

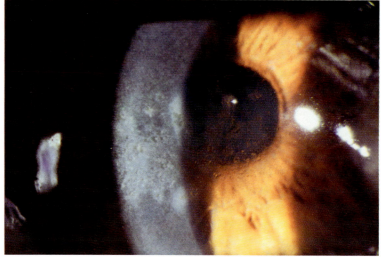

A

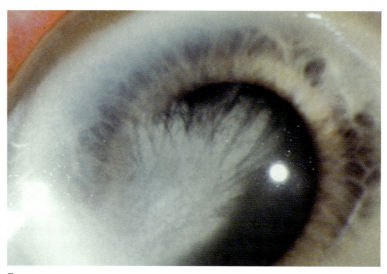

B

Figure 6-4   Spheroidal degeneration   A. *Gray and brown deposits are seen in the interpalpebral area. These can be mildly or moderately elevated.* **Lipid keratopathy   B.** *Creamy-white lipid deposits in the corneal stroma are apparent in a feathery pattern. The clearer lines are "ghost" vessels, areas of previous corneal neovascularization. (Continued.)*

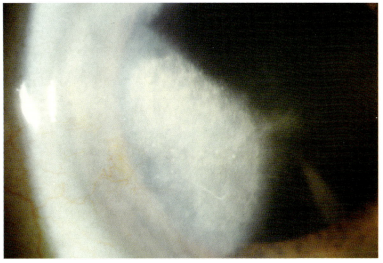

C

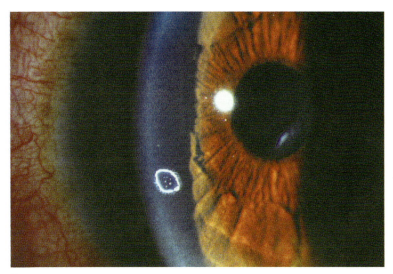

D

Figure 6-4 (cont.)   Lipid keratopathy   C. *White stromal lipid deposits in a crystalline pattern are noted central to an area of corneal neovascularization.* **Coats' white ring   D.** *This small, bright white oval ring is the result of a old metallic foreign body injury.*

CORNEAL DEPOSITS—PIGMENTED

CORNEA VERTICILLATA (VORTEX KERATOPATHY)

Cornea verticillata is a condition occurring in patients with Fabry's disease, but is found much more commonly due to a variety of drugs.

Etiology

Fabry's Disease   An X-linked recessive sphingolipidosis characterized by cornea verticillata, conjunctival aneurysms, lens opacities, papilledema, optic atrophy, and macular and retinal edema. Cornea verticillata is seen in males with Fabry's disease and the female carriers.

Drugs That Can Cause Cornea Verticillata
- Amiodarone (most common) (Figure 6-5)
- Chloroquine
- Hydroxychloroquine
- Chlorpromazine
- Indomethacin
- Atovaquone

Signs

- Bilateral, symmetrical, golden-brownish epithelial deposits arranged in a curvilinear fashion from a point below the pupil and swirling outward but sparing the limbus

Treatment

- As this disorder is asymptomatic, no treatment is required.

Prognosis

- Excellent. The drug-related deposits tend to resolve upon discontinuation of the medication.

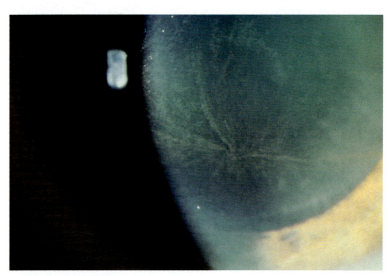

Figure 6-5   Cornea verticillata   *Superficial brown deposits appearing to emanate from a point in the inferior cornea are apparent in this patient taking amiodarone. These deposits do not affect vision. They eventually disappear upon discontinuation of the drug.*

CRYSTALLINE KERATOPATHY

Infectious Crystalline Keratopathy

- This is an uncommon condition, usually caused by indolent organisms such as *Streptococcus viridans*. Other bacteria and fungi can also cause this condition. It may develop as a complication of penetrating keratoplasty and/or the long-term use of topical corticosteroids.
- Discrete, white, branching crystalline deposits in the anterior stroma without significant associated inflammation are noted (Figure 6-6A).
- Treatment is with corneal cultures and intensive topical antibiotic therapy.

Other Causes of Corneal Crystals

Cystinosis Autosomal recessive condition resulting in deposits of the amino acid cystine in conjunctiva, corneal stroma, iris, lens, and retina, depending on severity. There may be growth retardation, renal failure, hepatosplenomegaly, and hypothyroidism (see Figures 8-3A,B).

Gout

Monoclonal Gammopathies Includes multiple myeloma, lymphoma, and Waldenstrom's macroglobulinemia.

Chrysiasis Deposits of gold particles in posterior corneal stroma and lens after chronic usage of gold-containing drugs for treatment of rheumatoid arthritis.

Argyrosis Deposition of silver-gray particles in posterior stroma as a result of long-term use of silver-containing drops.

Other Drugs Chloroquine, indomethacin, ciprofloxacin (Figure 6-6B).

Hyperlipidemia/Hypercholesterolemia
Schnyder's crystalline dystrophy (see Figures 5-8 A,B).

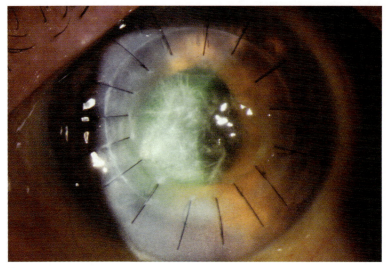

A

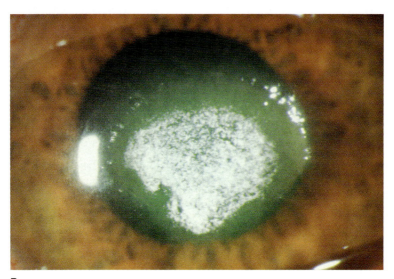

B

Figure 6-6 Infectious crystalline keratopathy **A.** *A crystalline, branching infiltrate is seen centrally in this corneal transplant. Culture revealed Streptococcus viridans.* **Ciprofloxacin deposits** **B.** *Confluent white deposits are seen in this cornea being treated with hourly ciprofloxacin drops for an infectious corneal ulcer. These deposits resolve as the epithelium heals and as the medication frequency is reduced.*

CORNEAL IRON DEPOSITS

Epithelial

Rust Ring   Consists of residual rust following the removal of a metallic foreign body.

Hudson Stahli's Line   Occurs at the junction of the upper two thirds and the lower third of an otherwise normal cornea.

Ferry's Line   Occurs in front of a filtering bleb.

Stocker's Line   Occurs in front of a pterygium.

Fleischer's Ring   Occurs at the base of the cone in keratoconus (see Figure 4-1C).

• Other iron lines may be found adjacent to corneal elevations in Salzmann's degeneration. (Figure 6-7A), corneal grafts, and after refractive surgery such as radial keratotomy (Figure 6-7B), PRK, and laser-assisted in-situ keratomileusis (LASIK).

Stromal

Siderosis   As a result of an intraocular iron foreign body

Corneal Blood Staining   Due to hyphema, especially an "eight-ball" hyphema. Clears slowly from the periphery (Figure 6-7C)

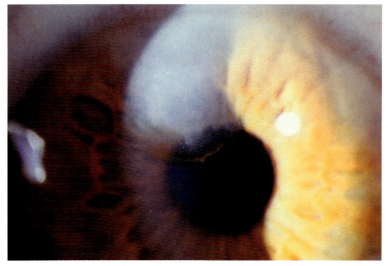

A

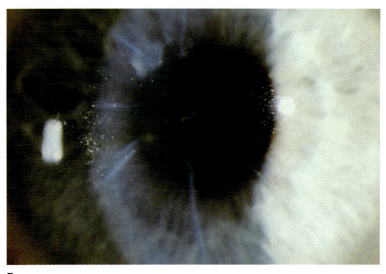

B

Figure 6-7 Iron line at the base of an elevated lesion A. *An iron line can be seen at the base of this longstanding elevated Salzmann's nodule.* **Iron line after refractive surgery** **B.** *A stellate iron line is present centrally in this eye with corneal flattening several years after radial keratotomy for myopia. (Continued.)*

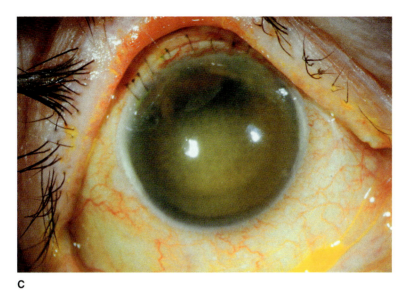

C

Figure 6-7 (cont.)   Corneal blood staining   C. *There is significant brown corneal stromal deposition in this eye. The patient had previously undergone an extracapsular cataract extraction and subsequent trauma resulting in dehiscence of the cataract wound and a total hyphema. The wound was repaired, but significant blood staining developed. Note there is some clearing of the blood staining from the periphery.*

KAYSER-FLEISCHER RING

- Bilateral, greenish-brown, peripheral band 1 to 3 mm in width at the level of Descemet's membrane, which occurs primarily in Wilson's disease.
- The band first appears in the vertical meridian, then extends to involve the entire corneal circumference. Early cases may require gonioscopy to visualize the deposits (Figure 6-8; see also Figure 8-1).
- May have associated subcapsular lenticular deposits resulting in a "sunflower" cataract in Wilson's disease.

Causes

- Wilson's disease (hepatolenticular degeneration): most common cause of a Kayser-Fleischer ring. A rare autosomal recessive condition caused by a deficiency of the enzyme ceruloplasmin. Characterized by liver cirrhosis and motor disorders. Treatment with copper chelating agents such as D-penicillamine or tetrathiomolybdate may improve the condition and be followed by resolution of corneal deposits.
- Primary biliary cirrhosis.
- Chronic active hepatitis.
- Multiple myeloma.

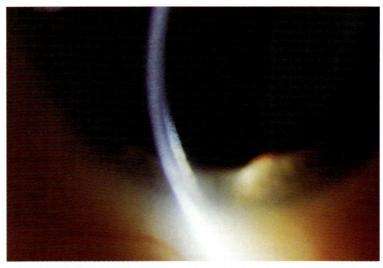

Figure 6-8 Kayser-Fleischer ring *Slit-lamp view of the inferior cornea of a patient with Wilson's disease. Note the brown pigment at the level of Descemet's membrane peripherally. In early cases, the pigment may be seen best using gonioscopy. See also* **Figure 8-1.**

TERRIEN'S MARGINAL DEGENERATION

Terrien's marginal degeneration is an uncommon, often bilateral, painless, slowly progressive peripheral corneal thinning condition.

Etiology

- Unknown. Affects males more commonly than females, generally in the second to fourth decades.

Symptoms

- Patients are asymptomatic with mild disease. More advanced disease causes decreased vision from severe against-the-rule astigmatism, which is commonly irregular.

Signs

- Noninflamed, peripheral thinning associated with a vascularized pannus and lipid deposits central to the thinned edge. The thinning usually begins superiorly and extends circumfer-entially, although it can begin inferiorly. Epithelium remains intact (Figures 6-9A,B).
- Perforation is rare and is usually associated with blunt trauma.

Treatment

- Mild cases can be treated with glasses or soft contact lenses. Moderate cases can achieve good vision with rigid gas-permeable contact lenses. Advanced cases may require a crescentic inlay lamellar keratoplasty for tectonic purposes.

Prognosis

- Good for mild and moderate disease. Fair for severe disease

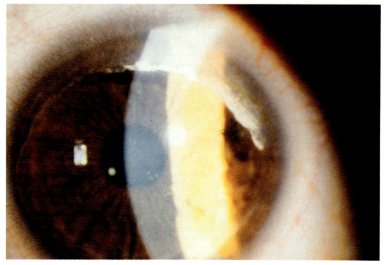

A

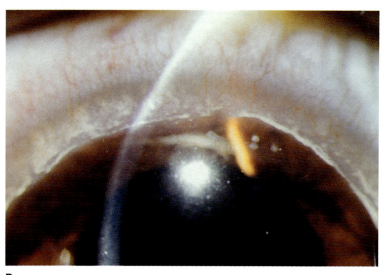

B

Figure 6-9 Terrien's marginal degeneration **A.** *Superior peripheral corneal thinning with overlying pannus is seen. A dense arc of lipid deposition is seen at the central edge of the thinning.* **B.** *Slit-lamp beam view reveals corneal thinning, pannus, and lipid deposition superiorly.*

IRIDOCORNEAL-ENDOTHELIAL (ICE) SYNDROME

ICE syndrome is a rare, unilateral, noninherited condition affecting the cornea, iris, and anterior chamber angle and is associated with glaucoma.

Etiology

- More common in young to middle-aged females
- ICE syndrome consists of three overlapping types: (1) essential iris atrophy—iris thinning, iris holes, corectopia, pseudopolycoria; (2) Chandler's syndrome—mild iris thinning and corectopia, marked corneal edema; (3) Cogan-Reese (iris nevus) syndrome—multiple small pigmented iris nodules

Histopathology Epithelioid metaplasia of corneal endothelium which can grow across the anterior chamber angle

Symptoms

- Asymptomatic in early stages. Cosmetic symptoms can result from iris changes. Decreased vision occurs from corneal edema and occasionally glaucoma.

Signs

- Common features include an abnormal corneal endothelium with a faintly hazy, beaten-metal appearance and broad peripheral anterior synechiae extending beyond Schwalbe's line (Figures 6-10A,B,C,D).
- Glaucoma results from synechial angle closure and is most severe in Chandler's syndrome.

Differential Diagnosis

- Axenfeld-Rieger syndrome: prominent anteriorly displaced Schwalbe's line, peripheral iris strands, possible systemic abnormalities
- Posterior polymorphous dystrophy: autosomal dominant and bilateral, more corneal and fewer iris changes

Treatment

- Treatment includes medical or surgical therapy to lower intraocular pressure and corneal transplantation for corneal decompensation.

Prognosis

- Good to very good if the glaucoma can be controlled. The glaucoma can be difficult to control without surgery and increases the risk of graft failure.

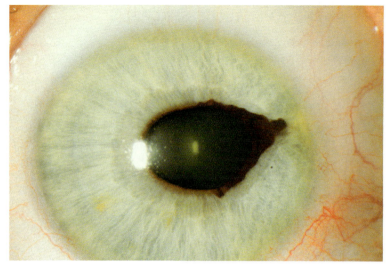

A

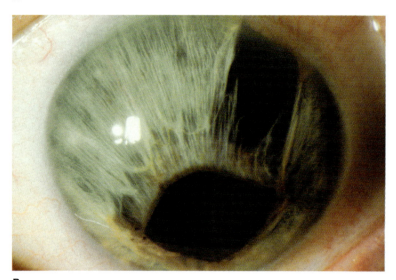

B

Figure 6-10   Iridocorneal-endothelial (ICE) syndrome   A. *This eye has mild essential iris atrophy. Note the ectropion uveae and corectopia.* **B.** *This eye has essential iris atrophy with peripheral anterior synechiae inferiorly and a large stretch hole superiorly. (Continued.)*

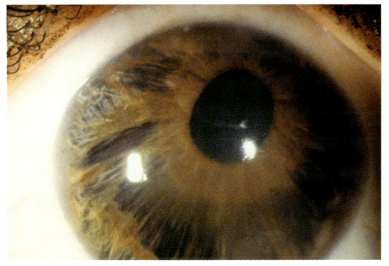

C

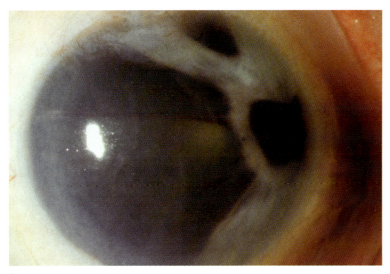

D

Figure 6-10 (cont.)   Iridocorneal-endothelial (ICE) syndrome   C. *There is an updrawn pupil due to progressive peripheral anterior synechiae formation superiorly and diffuse iris thinning in this eye with essential iris atrophy. Mild corneal edema is present.* **D.** *Severe corectopia with the pupil drawn toward the 3 o'clock limbus can be seen in this eye with essential iris atrophy. There are several large stretch holes. This patient underwent a corneal graft for severe corneal edema.*

Chapter 7

CORNEAL INFECTIONS, INFLAMMATIONS, AND SURFACE DISORDERS

BACTERIAL KERATITIS

Bacterial keratitis is a serious, potentially sight-threatening corneal infection which typically develops in patients with a compromised corneal surface.

Predisposing Factors

- Contact lens wear: especially extended-wear soft lenses
- Corneal trauma, foreign bodies
- Ocular surface disease (e.g., exposure/neurotrophic keratopathy, chronic bullous keratopathy, dry eye syndrome, trichiasis, distichiasis, entropion)
- Topical immunosuppressive therapy (e.g., corticosteroids)
- Immunocompromised patient
- Postoperative: corneal wound or suture-related (e.g., corneal graft)

Etiology

- *Staphylococcus*
- *Streptococcus*
- *Pseudomonas*
- *Moraxella*
- Atypical mycobacteria, others

Symptoms

- Pain, irritation, redness, photophobia, discharge, decreased vision, contact lens intolerance

Signs

- Vary according to the severity of the infection and, to a lesser extent, on the causative organism.
- White stromal infiltrate associated with conjunctival injection and typically with an overlying epithelial defect. There may be stromal loss (ulcer) (Figures 7-1A,B).
- There may be surrounding stromal edema, Descemet's folds, secondary reactive iritis, and hypopyon (Figures 7-1C,D).
- Staphylococcal keratitis is characterized by a well-defined, white-gray or creamy stromal infiltrate that may enlarge to form a dense stromal abscess.
- Streptococcal keratitis can be suppurative or have a crystalline appearance. Severe anterior uveitis and hypopyon formation are common.
- Pseudomonal keratitis presents as a rapidly progressive, suppurative infiltrate associated with hypopyon and a mucopurulent discharge. Corneal perforation may occur (Figure 7-1E).

Differential Diagnosis

- Sterile ulcers: vernal shield ulcer, neurotrophic or exposure keratitis, autoimmune keratitis, contact-lens induced sterile keratitis, medicamentosa keratitis. Usually less painful, minimal or no iritis or corneal edema and culture for bacteria is negative.
- Staphylococcal hypersensitivity keratitis: infiltrates may be bilateral; multiple; peripheral; located at 2, 4, 8, or 10 o'clock positions; associated with blepharitis; epithelial defect is absent or is smaller than the infiltrate; and there is minimal anterior chamber activity.
- Other microbial (nonbacterial) keratitis: bacterial cultures are negative. Fungal and special cultures and stains are necessary for diagnosis.

Diagnosis

- Corneal scraping for Gram's stain, Giemsa stain, calcofluor white stain, cultures, and sensitivity testing. Routine media include blood, chocolate, Sabouraud's agars, and thioglycolate broths.
- For deep lesions or when repeated cultures are negative in recalcitrant cases, a corneal biopsy may be necessary.

Treatment

- Empirical outpatient treatment with broad-spectrum, topical, nonfortified antibiotic drops may be sufficient for small (2 mm or less) peripheral ulcers with minimal symptoms and minimal anterior chamber activity. Topical fluoroquinolone (e.g., levofloxacin, ciprofloxacin, or ofloxacin) drops q 30 to 60 min around the clock initially after a loading dose of 1 drop q 5 min for 15 min.

- For larger ulcers or when the ulcers involve the visual axis, or are associated with significant discharge, anterior chamber activity, and hypopyon, treatment may require intensive fortified antibiotic drops. Patients are often hospitalized. Fortified cefazolin (50 mg/mL) or vancomycin (25 mg/mL) *and* fortified gentamicin or tobramycin (15 mg/mL). Frequency of instillation: 1 drop q 5 min for 30 min, then q 30 to 60 min for 24 hours of each drop. Wait 5 minutes between administration of each medication.
- Subconjunctival antibiotics are only necessary if fortified eye drops cannot be started soon.
- Oral antibiotics (e.g., ciprofloxacin 500 mg bid or levofloxacin 500 mg qd) are helpful when the ulcer involves the sclera or has extended into the eye. Systemic antibiotics are also required for *Neisseria* and *Haemophilus* infection (e.g., ceftriaxone 1 g IV or IM q 12 to 24 h).
- Cycloplegics are often used to reduce ciliary spasm and to prevent posterior synechiae (e.g., scopolamine 0.25% or atropine 1% tid).
- Modify regimen according to clinical response and culture and sensitivity results.
- Topical corticosteroids can be used for severe inflammation only after the organism is identified and the infection is under control.
- Corneal graft may be necessary in severe cases that are progressing despite aggressive treatment or for ulcers that have perforated.

Prognosis

- Close follow-up is required. Prognosis is very good for small ulcers, good for moderate ulcers, poor for severe ulcers. Better prognosis for ulcers outside the visual axis than ulcers in the visual axis.

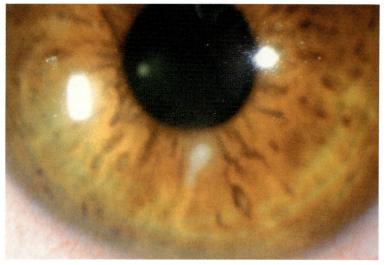

A

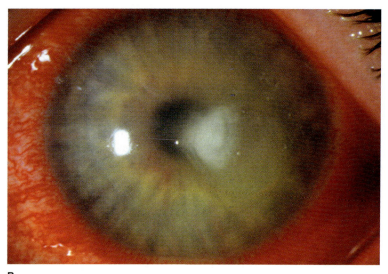

B

Figure 7-1   Bacterial keratitis   A. *This small inferior corneal infiltrate in an overnight soft contact lens wearer has some underlying corneal edema. Because it may be an early infectious keratitis, it should be treated with topical antibiotics and followed closely.* **B.** *This dense central corneal ulcer has a large overlying epithelial defect and moderate underlying corneal edema. There is a small hypopyon inferiorly. (Continued.)*

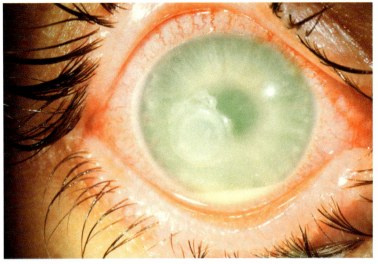

C

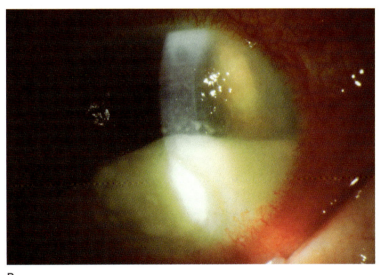

D

Figure 7-1 (cont.) **Bacterial keratitis** **C.** *This corneal infection was due to Pseudomonas aeruginosa. There is a large circular corneal ulcer with overlying mucopurulent discharge, underlying corneal edema and a moderately large hypopyon.* **D.** *This large dense corneal ulcer is associated with a hypopyon that fills approximately 50% of the anterior chamber. (Continued.)*

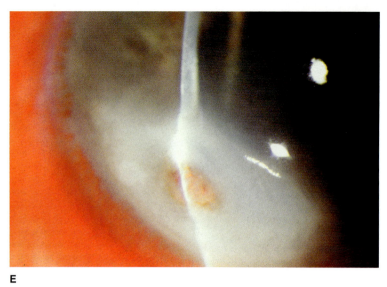

E

Figure 7-1 (cont.) **Bacterial keratitis** **E.** *This infected corneal ulcer caused a perforation. Iris is plugging the wound. The anterior chamber is shallow but formed.*

FUNGAL KERATITIS

Fungal keratitis is a very serious, potentially sight-threatening corneal infection which most commonly develops in patients after trauma or those with a compromised corneal surface.

Etiology

Nonfilamentous (e.g., *Candida*) *Candida* keratitis is a rare, unilateral, insidious fungal infection that usually occurs in eyes with pre-existing chronic corneal disease (e.g., dry eyes, herpes keratitis, exposure keratopathy, postkeratoplasty, chronic use of corticosteroid drops) or in severely debilitated patients. Features include a gray-white stromal infiltrate similar to a bacterial ulcer. May have an anterior chamber reaction and hypopyon (Figures 7-2A,B).

Filamentous (e.g., *Aspergillus*, *Fusarium*, etc.) Filamentous keratitis is a rare, unilateral, insidious fungal infection that frequently affects normal eyes following ocular trauma associated with vegetative matter and in soft contact lens wearers. Features include a grayish-white infiltrate with indistinct feathery borders, typically surrounded by finger-like satellite infiltrates in adjacent stroma. The infiltrates may extend beyond the epithelial defect. May have an associated ring infiltrate, anterior chamber reaction, and hypopyon (Figures 7-2C,D).

Symptoms

- Pain, photophobia, tearing, decreased vision; may have a history of trauma or corticosteroid eye drop usage

Differential Diagnosis

- Fungal keratitis should be considered in the differential diagnosis of bacterial or herpetic keratitis that does not respond to conventional treatment or has an unusual history or suspicious appearance.

Diagnosis

- History of trauma (which is often minor) involving vegetative matter is highly suggestive.
- Lack of response to conventional antibacterial therapy.
- Corneal scrapings for Giemsa, calcofluor white, or Gomori methenamine silver stain, and culture (may take up to a week for fungus to grow).
- Corneal biopsy may be required if smears and cultures are negative.

Treatment

- Topical natamycin 5% (especially for filamentous fungi) and/or amphotericin B 0.15% (especially for *Candida*) q 1 h around the clock and taper over 4 to 6 weeks. Patients are often hospitalized initially.
- Oral itraconazole or fluconazole 200 to 400 mg loading dose followed by 100 to 200 mg qd.
- Cycloplegics (e.g., scopolamine 0.25% or atropine 1% tid).
- Corticosteroids are contraindicated.
- Epithelial debridement may facilitate topical therapy by enhancing penetration of antifungals.
- Modify regimen according to clinical response and culture results.
- Therapeutic penetrating keratoplasty may be necessary for unresponsive cases or perforated ulcers. Lamellar keratoplasty is discouraged as there is a high risk of recurrence of infection.

Prognosis

- Fair for mild to moderate infections. Poor for severe infections.

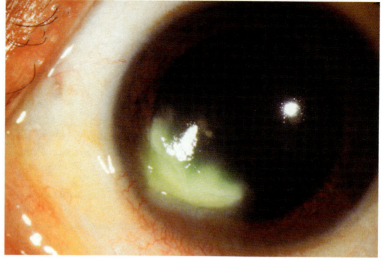

A

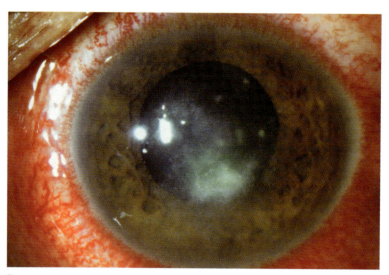

B

Figure 7-2 Fungal keratitis A. *This multilobulated dense infiltrate was caused by a Candida infection. There is an overlying epithelial defect. Peripheral corneal neovascularization suggests it is a long-standing ulcer.* **B.** *This Candida corneal ulcer is slowly improving. The denser infiltrate at the inferior pupillary margin is surrounded by multiple satellite lesions. (Continued.)*

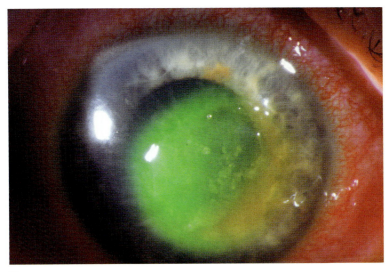

C

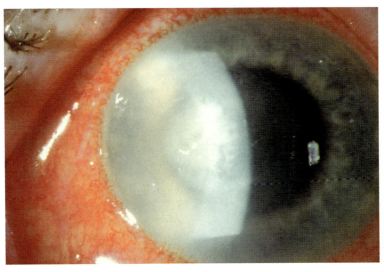

D

Figure 7-2 (cont.)   Fungal keratitis   C. *This multicentric corneal ulcer was caused by Fusarium. There is a large epithelial defect with significant underlying corneal edema.* **D.** *This dense white infiltrate with feathery borders was due to a Fusarium infection. A ring infiltrate is beginning inferiorly.*

ACANTHAMOEBA KERATITIS

Acanthamoeba keratitis is a rare parasitic infection of the cornea associated with the use of soft contact lenses and inadequate contact lens hygiene (e.g., using tap water or homemade saline solutions, swimming or hot tub use while wearing contact lenses). It should be considered in nonhealing, culture-negative keratitis.

Etiology

- *Acanthamoeba* species

Symptoms

- Severe pain out of proportion to severity of keratitis, redness, tearing, decreased vision, photophobia, minimal discharge. Symptoms typically develop over a period of weeks, but onset can be more rapid.
- History of soft contact lens use and occasionally trauma.

Signs

- Epithelial or subepithelial infiltrates appearing as pseudodendrites early on (Figure 7-3A).
- A nonsuppurative stromal ring infiltrate often with variable epithelial breakdown can develop over weeks. The degree of inflammation is disproportionate to the amount of pain (Figures 7-3B,C).
- Radial keratoneuritis.
- In advanced cases, corneal thinning or perforation, scleritis, or hypopyon may develop.

Differential Diagnosis

- Herpes simplex keratitis
- Fungal keratitis
- Bacterial keratitis

Diagnosis

- Pain disproportionate to severity of inflammation.
- Lack of response to antibacterial and antiviral therapy.

- Ring infiltrate and radial keratoneuritis are highly suggestive.
- Corneal scrapings for Gram's, Giemsa, or calcofluor white stain for amoebic cysts.
- Culture on non-nutrient agar with *E. coli* overlay or special media (e.g., buffered charcoal yeast extract agar).
- Corneal biopsy may be necessary if smears and cultures are negative.

Treatment

- Propamidine isethionate 1% (e.g., Brolene®) drops q 1 h.
- Neomycin-polymyxin B-gramicidin (e.g. Neosporin®) drops q 1 h.
- Polyhexamethylene biguanide (PHMB) 0.02% drops q 1 h. Chlorhexidine 0.02% can be used as an alternative to PHMB.
- Oral itraconazole 100 to 200 mg qd or ketoconazole 200 mg qd.
- Other drops (e.g., clotrimazole) may be added depending on severity or treatment response of the infection.
- Cycloplegics (e.g., scopolamine 0.25% or atropine 1% tid).
- Low-dose topical corticosteroids may be helpful in reducing inflammation.
- Oral nonsteroidal anti-inflammatory agents or narcotics for pain relief.
- Modify regimen according to clinical response.
- Penetrating keratoplasty may be required if medical therapy fails, but there is risk of recurrence.

Prognosis

- Fair to good if diagnosed and treated appropriately within the first month of development of symptoms. Poor if significant corneal involvement is present.

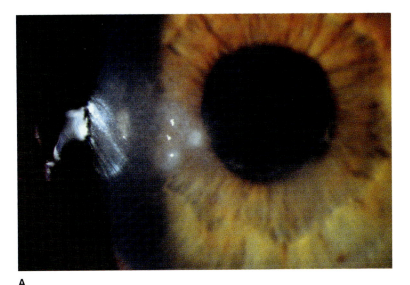

A

B

Figure 7-3 Acanthamoeba keratitis A. *This early* Acanthamoeba *infection has several subepithelial infiltrates in a linear pattern reminiscent of a dendrite, hence the term pseudodendrite. There was no frank epithelial defect, but there was epithelial irregularity* **B.** *After several weeks, a ring infiltrate can develop, as can be seen especially superiorly. There is a small epithelial defect inferocentrally. (Continued.)*

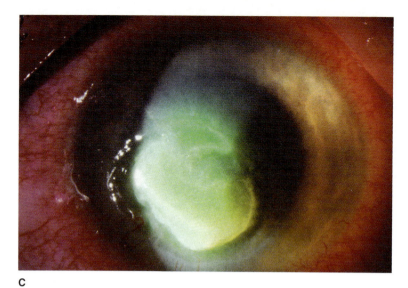

C

Figure 7-3 (cont.)   Acanthamoeba keratitis   C. *After several months of antiacanthamoeba treatment, this dense infiltrate is finally scarring. The active infection eventually resolved but the eye was left with a significant corneal scar.*

HERPES SIMPLEX KERATITIS (HSV)

Herpes simplex infection is an extremely common condition affecting a major proportion of the population, although most infections are subclinical. The eyes can be affected in primary ocular herpes or in recurrent disease.

Etiology

Herpes Simplex Virus Type 1 Causes infection above the waist, especially the face, lips, and eyes. Transmitted by close contact. Much more common in the eye.

Herpes Simplex VirusType 2 Causes infection below the waist, particularly the genitalia. Transmitted sexually, but neonates can be infected during vaginal delivery. Uncommon in the eye.

PRIMARY OCULAR HERPES

- Unilateral or bilateral facial and/or eye infection

Etiology and Epidemiology

- Primary contact with HSV
- Usually occurs in children or adolescents

Symptoms

- Fever, flu-like symptoms
- Facial vesicular rash. Ocular redness, pain, decreased vision, and tearing

Signs

- There may be vesicular blepharoconjunctivitis or periorbital dermatitis. The vesicles usually progress to form crusts (Figures 7-4A,B). There may be associated acute follicular conjunctivitis with preauricular lymphadenopathy.
- The cornea may be involved in the form of coarse macropunctate epithelial keratitis or multiple small branching epithelial dendrites without stromal involvement.

Treatment

Blepharoconjunctivitis Vidarabine (e.g., Vira-A®) ointment, trifluridine (e.g., Viroptic®) drops, or acyclovir (e.g., Zovirax® ophthalmic) ointment 5 times a day.

Corneal Involvement Trifluridine drops (e.g., Viroptic) 9 times a day.

- Consider acyclovir 200 to 400 mg po 5 times a day for 7 to 14 days.
- Consider topical antibiotic ointment or acyclovir to help heal skin lesions away from the eyelid margin.

Prognosis

- Good. This is usually a benign and self-limited condition, but the virus subsequently establishes a latent infection in the trigeminal ganglion and may reactivate, especially during periods of physical or emotional stress, to cause recurrent disease.

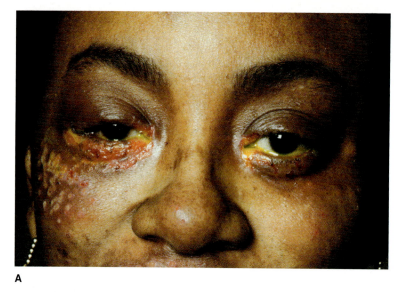

A

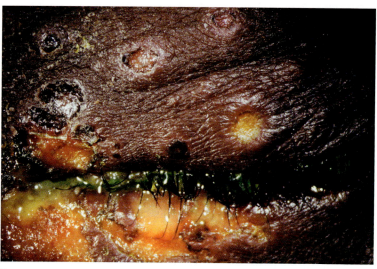

B

Figure 7-4   Herpes simplex dermatitis   A. *This patient had recurrent herpes simplex dermatitis. Note the numerous ulcerated skin lesions around the right eye and cheek. The right eye appears uninvolved, but should receive prophylactic treatment due to skin lesions on the eyelid margin.* **B.** *Multiple ulcerated skin lesions of herpes simplex can be seen in the upper eyelid. Confluent skin ulcerations are present in the lower eyelid with a mucoid discharge.*

RECURRENT OCULAR HERPES SIMPLEX

Recurrent ocular herpes may take the form of infectious epithelial keratitis, non-necrotizing stromal keratitis (disciform keratitis), necrotizing stromal keratitis, neurotrophic keratitis, and keratouveitis.

Etiology and Epidemiology

- Recurrent HSV is due to a reactivation of latent infection in the trigeminal ganglion, especially during periods of physical or emotional stress.
- It occurs in children and adults.

HSV: EPITHELIAL KERATITIS (DENDRITIC ULCER)

Epithelial keratitis is a very common, usually unilateral condition due to the presence of live virus within corneal epithelial cells.

Symptoms

- Unilateral redness, tearing, irritation, decreased vision, photophobia, history of previous episodes

Signs

- Single or multiple branching, ulcerating epithelial lesions with raised edges and terminal bulb formation (Figures 7-5A,B).
- Enlargement of ulcers can lead to the formation of an amebic-shaped geographic ulcer.
- The ulcer bed stains with fluorescein. The built-up, swollen, opalescent margins of the lesion containing virus-laden cells stain with rose bengal.
- Anterior stromal haze called "ghost dendrites" may develop below the epithelial lesions (Figure 7-5C).
- Corneal sensation may be diminished.

Differential Diagnosis

- Herpes zoster keratitis: associated with herpes zoster ophthalmicus with typical skin vesicles found along dermatomal distribution of the face. May have elevated epithelial lesions with tapered ends, which lack terminal bulbs. The entire lesion stains with rose bengal and mildly with fluorescein. Prior to development of the typical zoster rash, early zoster dendrites can look very similar to HSV dendrites.
- *Acanthamoeba* pseudodendrites.
- Healing epithelial defects.
- Toxic epitheliopathy.

Treatment

- Trifluridine (e.g., Viroptic) drops q 2 h during the day or vidarabine (e.g., Vira-A) or acyclovir (e.g., Zovirax ophthalmic) ointment 5 times a day.
- If the patient is already on corticosteroids, they should be tapered rapidly.
- Epithelial debridement can help reduce viral load.
- If there is no response to treatment after 1 week, then poor compliance, resistance to antiviral therapy, antiviral toxicity, or neurotrophic disease should be considered.
- A short course of systemic acyclovir is unnecessary as it does not prevent subsequent development of stromal keratitis or uveitis, but can be used when frequent topical antivirals cannot be given.
- Consider long-term oral antiviral prophylaxis (e.g., acyclovir 400 mg bid) if a patient has had multiple episodes of herpetic eye disease.

Prognosis

- Good. Recurrences are common.

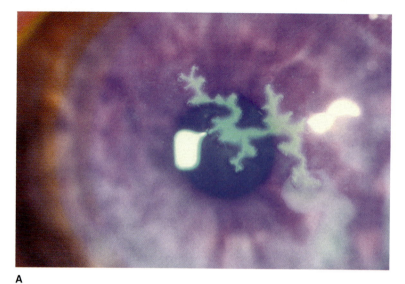

A

B

Figure 7-5 Herpes simplex keratitis A. *Fluorescein staining with a cobalt blue light of an active herpes simplex epithelial dendrite. Note the "tree branching" pattern of the dendrite. The central bed stains well with fluorescein while the elevated edges do not. The ends of the dendrite have classic terminal "end bulbs." **B.** Rose bengal dye on this active dendrite stains the built-up edges which contain virus-laden cells. (Continued.)*

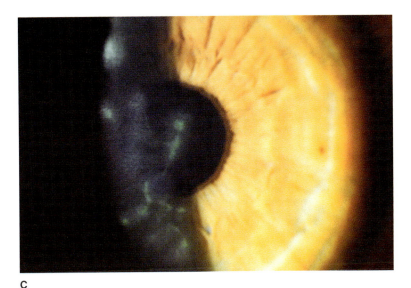

C

Figure 7-5 (cont.)   Herpes simplex keratitis   C. *This resolving epithelial dendrite barely stains with fluorescein. There is residual underlying corneal haze in the pattern of the previous dendrite, often termed a "ghost dendrite."*

HSV: NON-NECROTIZING STROMAL KERATITIS (DISCIFORM KERATITIS)

Disciform keratitis is a primarily inflammatory condition caused by a hypersensitivity reaction to the herpes simplex viral antigen in the cornea.

Symptoms

- Unilateral redness, tearing, irritation, blurred vision, photophobia, history of previous episodes

Signs

- Central disc of stromal and epithelial edema (Figure 7-6A).
- Small keratic precipitates localized to the underlying endothelium.
- Folds in Descemet's membrane.
- Surrounding stromal immune ring (Wessley ring) may be present.
- The limbal tissue may be thickened and inflamed (limbitis) (Figure 7-6B).
- Anterior uveitis (Figures 7-6C,D).
- Intraocular pressure may be elevated.
- Corneal sensation is typically reduced.

Differential Diagnosis

- Acute corneal hydrops of keratoconus
- Fuchs' endothelial dystrophy
- Herpes zoster disciform keratitis
- Contact lens overwear

Treatment

- If inflammation is mild and vision is good, the condition can be observed.
- In more severe cases, topical corticosteroids (e.g., prednisolone 1%, dexamethasone 0.1%, or loteprednol 0.5% drops qid) can be started, maintained for several days to weeks, then gradually tapered over weeks or months. Often, a very low dose (once or twice a week) may be required to prevent recurrent inflammation.
- While on corticosteroids more than once a day, concomitant antiviral drops (qid) or ointment (bid) is often required as prophylaxis.
- If an epithelial lesion is present, it should be treated before starting corticosteroids.
- Consider long-term oral antiviral prophylaxis (e.g., acyclovir 400 mg bid) if a patient has had multiple episodes of stromal keratitis.

Prognosis

- Good. Stromal scarring may occur and reduce vision (Figure 7-6E). Often recurs.

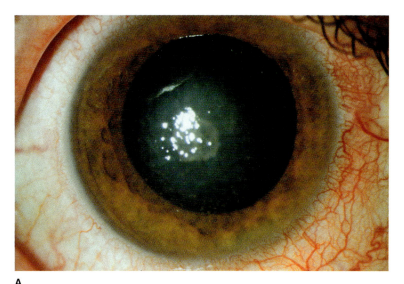

A

B

Figure 7-6 Herpes simplex disciform keratitis A. *This eye has severe central corneal edema with underlying keratic precipitates. This disciform keratitis represents an inflammatory reaction to previous herpes simplex infection. It may resolve spontaneously, but often responds extremely well to topical corticosteroids with antiviral coverage.* **Herpes simplex limbitis B.** *This eye, with a previous history of herpes simplex keratitis, has severe limbal inflammation. Note the thickened, elevated limbal conjunctiva. This limbitis responded to topical corticosteroids and antiviral coverage. (Continued.)*

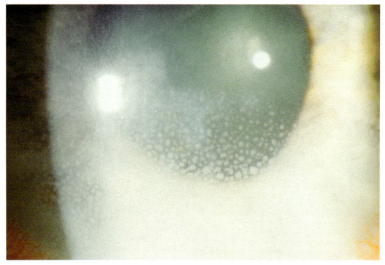

C

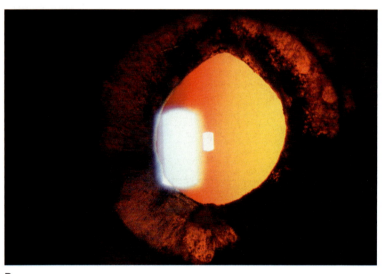

D

Figure 7-6 (cont.)   Herpes simplex iritis   C. *Hundreds of granulomatous keratic precipitates are present in this eye with a history of previous herpes simplex keratitis. Note the faint central corneal scarring of old herpes keratitis. Often the intraocular pressure is elevated in eyes with herpetic iritis. Herpes simplex iritis responds to topical corticosteroids with antiviral coverage. It likely benefits from treatment with oral antiviral agents in addition.* **Herpes simplex keratitis   D.** *Retroillumination off the retina reveals significant iris stromal atrophy and iris transillumination defects after multiple episodes of herpes simplex keratitis and iritis. (Continued.)*

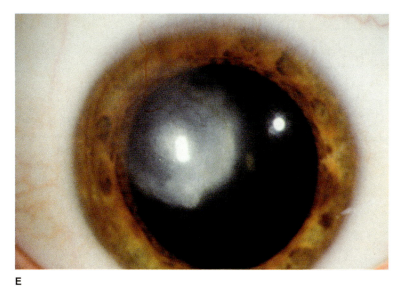

E

Figure 7-6 (cont.) Herpes simplex keratitis E. *A large dense corneal scar with neovascularization remains after repeated episodes of herpes simplex keratitis.*

HSV: NECROTIZING STROMAL KERATITIS

Necrotizing stromal keratitis is unusual. It is most likely caused by viral infiltration and inflammation of the corneal stroma.

Symptoms

- Unilateral redness, tearing, irritation, blurred vision, photophobia, pain, history of previous episodes.

Signs

- Necrotic, cheesy, stromal infiltration which may be associated with an epithelial defect (Figure 7-7A).
- The appearance of the infiltrate can be confused with secondary bacterial or fungal keratitis.
- Corneal thinning, stromal neovascularization, scarring or perforation may develop (Figure 7-7B).
- There may be associated keratic precipitates, anterior uveitis, or hypopyon.
- Intraocular pressure can be elevated even in the presence of minimal anterior chamber reaction.

Differential Diagnosis

- Primary or secondary bacterial or fungal keratitis: there is generally an overlying epithelial defect. These conditions should be considered when there is lack of response to antiviral treatment, and when there are increased or new signs of infection and inflammation.

Treatment

- The first priority is to treat any associated epithelial defect with antibiotic drops or ointment.
- Once the epithelium has healed, topical corticosteroids can be judiciously added to reduce stromal and anterior chamber inflammation (e.g., prednisolone 1% or dexamethasone 0.1% drops qid), combined with topical antiviral/antibacterial prophylaxis.
- Corticosteroid drops should be tapered gradually (strength and frequency) over weeks or months depending on the level of inflammation and the therapeutic response.
- Cycloplegics (e.g., scopolamine 0.25% or cyclopentolate 1% tid).
- Treat any elevated intraocular pressure. Avoid miotics and prostaglandin analogues.
- Systemic acyclovir may be helpful, especially when there is anterior uveitis (acyclovir 400 mg 5 times a day for weeks to months).
- Corneal transplant during acute stages of the infection is discouraged due to high failure rates.
- Recommend long-term oral antiviral prophylaxis (e.g., acyclovir 400 mg bid) if a patient has had past episodes of herpes stromal keratitis.

Prognosis

- Fair. Typically, significant stromal scarring remains, and if in the visual axis, can severely affect vision.

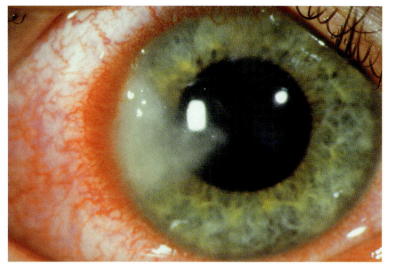

A

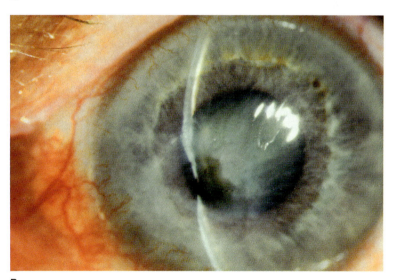

B

Figure 7-7   Herpes simplex necrotizing keratitis   **A.** *A necrotizing stromal keratitis can be seen from the 8 o'clock to 10 o'clock positions, reaching into the visual axis. A prominent limbitis is present. Old stromal scarring is present superiorly and centrally.* **B.** *This necrotizing herpes simplex keratitis caused a full thickness corneal melt and perforation. This large perforation required an emergent penetrating keratoplasty.*

HSV: NEUROTROPHIC KERATITIS (METAHERPETIC KERATITIS)

Neurotrophic keratitis is not due to active viral infection but is a healing problem caused by a combination of decreased sensation, drug toxicity, and a damaged basement membrane from epithelial infection due to herpes.

Symptoms

- Unilateral redness, tearing, irritation, blurred vision, photophobia, history of previous episodes.

Signs

- Persistent epithelial defect with heaped-up borders. The edges do not stain well with rose bengal. The base stains readily with fluorescein (Figure 7-8).
- There may be mild to moderate corneal haze.
- Epithelial dendrites and terminal bulbs are absent.
- May progress to corneal melting and perforation, especially if also using topical corticosteroids.
- Decreased corneal sensation.
- Reactive iritis may be present.

Differential Diagnosis

- Geographic herpes simplex ulcer: edges have branching dendritic extensions and stain well with rose bengal.

Treatment

- Discontinue toxic topical medications.
- Other measures to heal the epithelium are similar to those for neurotrophic keratopathy (see section on Neurotrophic Keratopathy).

Prognosis

- Good for small lesions, fair for large lesions. Often corneal haze/scar remains after the epithelial defect resolves.

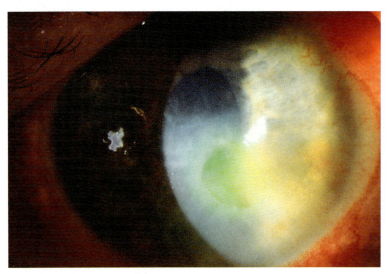

Figure 7-8 Herpes simplex neurotrophic keratitis *A neurotrophic corneal ulcer is present is this eye with recent herpes simplex keratitis. The active herpes infection was treated with topical antiviral agents and the active dendrite resolved. However, the epithelial defect remained, causing stromal thinning. Note the heaped up edges of epithelium.*

HERPES ZOSTER KERATITIS (HZV)

Herpes zoster infection is caused by a reactivation of the chickenpox virus in the dorsal root ganglion that has migrated down along the sensory nerves to affect the skin of that particular dermatome. When the ophthalmic division (V_1) of the trigeminal nerve is involved, the condition is called herpes zoster ophthalmicus.

Etiology and Epidemiology

- Varicella zoster virus.
- Unlike chickenpox, it is rare in children and typically affects elderly patients, but can also affect younger adults, especially those who are immunocompromised (e.g., HIV, cancer).

Symptoms

- Fever, malaise, and headache, which may precede the rash by a few days. May be difficult to diagnose during the prodromal stage
- Dermatomal skin rash, tingling, burning, itching sensation, pain
- Eye redness, irritation, tearing, decreased vision, photophobia

Signs

- Unilateral vesicular skin rash that does not cross the midline (Figure 7-9A). The rash subsequently forms blisters and crusts which heal with scarring. Hutchinson's sign, vesicles on the tip of the nose, indicates presence of nasociliary nerve involvement and may predict a higher risk of ocular disease.
- Periocular dermatitis, conjunctivitis, episcleritis, scleritis.
- Corneal involvement includes superficial punctate keratitis, microdendritic keratitis, nummular keratitis, disciform keratitis, and neurotrophic keratitis. Neurotrophic ulcers and persistent epithelial defects can lead to secondary infection, thinning, and eventually, corneal perforation (Figure 7-9B).
- Zoster pseudodendrites are elevated, "stuck-on" mucous-plaque lesions that stain with rose bengal but do not stain well with fluorescein and do not have terminal end bulbs (Figures 7-9C,D).
- Iritis, glaucoma, retinitis, optic neuritis, cranial nerve palsy, and cranial arteritis may be seen.
- Postherpetic neuralgia may also be present.

Differential Diagnosis

- Herpes simplex keratitis: patients are generally younger, have a history of recurrent episodes, involvement has no dermatomal distribution, dendrites have terminal bulbs, and the central parts are depressed and stain well with fluorescein.

Treatment

Skin Involvement

- Oral acyclovir 800 mg 5 times a day or fam-ciclovir 500 mg tid or valacyclovir 1000 mg tid for 7 to 10 days to be started as soon as possible
- H₂ antagonist (e.g., cimetidine 400 mg bid po) may reduce itching and pain
- Antiviral (e.g., acyclovir) and/or antibacterial (e.g., tetracycline, bacitracin, or erythromycin) ointment qid to the skin

Conjunctivitis, Episcleritis

- These are self-limited and treatment is for symptomatic relief.
- Cool compresses, artificial tears, or antibiotic ointment (e.g., erythromycin, bacitracin, or tetracycline) bid or tid.

Scleritis Consider oral nonsteroidal anti-inflammatory agents (e.g., flurbiprofen 100 mg tid) or corticosteroids (e.g., prednisolone 1 mg/kg/d qd for 2 weeks then taper) in severe cases.

Disciform Keratitis Topical corticosteroids in more severe cases (e.g., prednisolone 1%, dexamethasone 0.1%, or loteprednol 0.5% 4 to 8 times a day). Taper slowly. A very low dose may be required chronically to prevent recurrences.

Pseudodendrites

- Generally self-limited and treated with lubrication with artificial tear drops or ointment
- May respond to topical antiviral agents (e.g., vidarabine ointment), especially if immunocompromised

Neurotrophic Keratitis (see Section on Neurotrophic Keratopathy)

Retinitis, Choroiditis, Optic Neuritis Intravenous acyclovir and oral corticosteroids

Postherpetic Neuralgia Topical capsaicin or doxepin creams and/or systemic antidepressant medication may be helpful. In severe cases, referral to a neurologist or pain specialist is indicated.

All Patients

- Control iritis with topical corticosteroids.
- Control glaucoma. Beware of corticosteroid-induced pressure rise as a possible cause.

Prognosis

- Good to poor depending on the severity of the corneal involvement (Figure 7-9E). Chronic recurrent bouts of ocular inflammation are common. Postherpetic neuralgia can devastating in some patients.

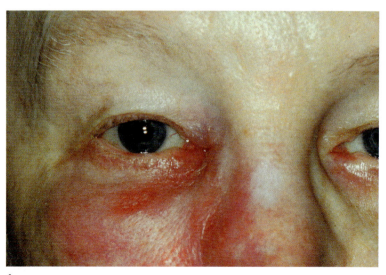

A

Figure 7-9 Herpes zoster dermatitis **A.** *A herpes zoster dermatitis (shingles) infection in the V₂ distribution. Note the ulcerated skin vesicles. (Continued.)*

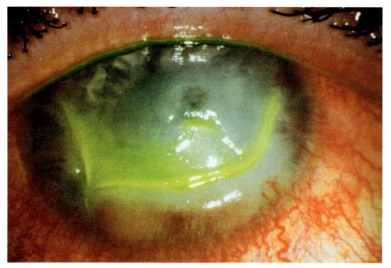

B

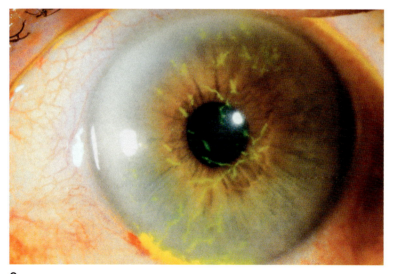

C

Figure 7-9 (cont.) Herpes zoster keratitis **B.** *Significant limbal inflammation and an active corneal melt are present in this eye with a history of herpes zoster keratitis. It responded well to a conjunctival flap procedure.* **C.** *Multiple elevated, plaquelike pseudodendrites are present in this eye several weeks after a herpes zoster dermatitis around this eye. (Continued.)*

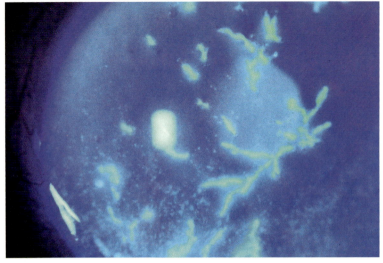

D

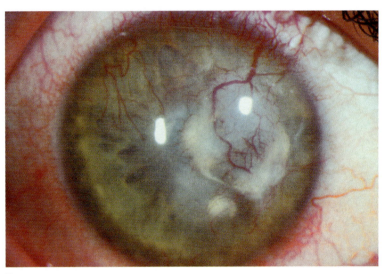

E

Figure 7-9 (cont.) **Herpes zoster keratitis** **D.** *Fluorescein stain with a cobalt blue light highlights the pseudodendrites seen in* **Figure 7-9C**. *Note that they lack the classic "tree branch" pattern, elevated edges and terminal end bulbs of herpes simplex dendrites.* **E.** *Eight years after an episode of herpes zoster ophthalmicus, there is significant corneal neovascularization and scarring. There is also some white lipid keratopathy surrounding the largest blood vessels.*

INTERSTITIAL KERATITIS (SYPHILITIC, NONSYPHILITIC)

Interstitial keratitis is an uncommon, bilateral inflammation of the corneal stroma without primary involvement of the epithelium or endothelium. It has a wide variety of causes.

Etiology

- Congenital or acquired syphilis (*Treponema pallidum*)
- Lyme disease (*Borrelia burgdorferi*)
- Tuberculosis (*Mycobacterium tuberculosis*)
- Herpes simplex, herpes zoster, Epstein-Barr, Mumps virus
- Leprosy (*Mycobacterium leprae*)
- Cogan's syndrome: tinnitus, vertigo, and deafness. Associated with polyarteritis nodosa, Wegener's granulomatosis, and rheumatoid arthritis. Rare.

Symptoms

- Bilateral pain, redness, tearing, blurred vision

Nonspecific Corneal Features

- Diffuse midstromal edema, neovascularization, and nonsuppurative infiltration
- Mild iritis, keratic precipitates
- Inactive signs include deep stromal scarring associated with nonperfused (ghost) vessels (Figures 7-10A,B)

Specific Ocular Features

Syphilis
- Congenital syphilis is associated with acute interstitial keratitis in the first two decades of life.
- Acquired syphilis has fewer corneal findings and more posterior segment involvement.

Tuberculosis   Interstitial keratitis, phlyctenulosis, granulomatous iridocyclitis, retinal vasculitis, choroiditis

Lyme Disease   Enlarging skin rash (erythema chronicum migrans), conjunctivitis, episcleritis, interstitial keratitis (Figure 7-10C), granulomatous iridocyclitis, intermediate uveitis, cranial nerve, retinal and orbital abnormalities

Leprosy   Conjunctivitis, episcleritis, scleritis, interstitial keratitis, thickened corneal nerves, corneal hypesthesia, granulomatous iridocyclitis, iris pearls, nodular leproma, iris atrophy, anisocoria, eyelid and lacrimal abnormalities, cataract, facial nerve palsy

Diagnosis

Syphilis
- Fluorescent treponemal antibody absorption (FTA-Abs) or microhemagglutination- *Treponema pallidum* (MHA-TP) test (specific tests for treponemal antibodies). Usually remains positive for life.
- Venereal Disease Research Laboratory (VDRL) or rapid plasma reagin (RPR) test (nonspecific tests are positive during acute infection). Useful for screening and for monitoring activity of disease.

Tuberculosis Examination of sputum for acid-fast bacilli, chest x-ray, purified protein derivative (PPD) skin test

Lyme Disease History of exposure to deer, mouse, or tick bite, direct immunofluorescent antibody test

Leprosy Skin scrapings for Ziehl-Neelsen stain

Cogan's Syndrome Consult an otorhinolaryngologist

Treatment

Keratouveitis Topical corticosteroids (prednisolone 1% or dexamethasone 0.1% q 2 to 4 h) and cycloplegics (scopolamine 0.25% or cyclopentolate 1% tid).

Syphilis, Tuberculosis, Lyme Disease, Leprosy Refer to an internist, pulmonologist, or infectious disease specialist for appropriate treatment.

Cogan's Syndrome Refer to an otorhinolaryngologist for systemic corticosteroid treatment to prevent permanent hearing loss.

Prognosis

- Generally good with appropriate treatment. Significant permanent corneal scarring can result and may require corneal transplantation when noninflamed.

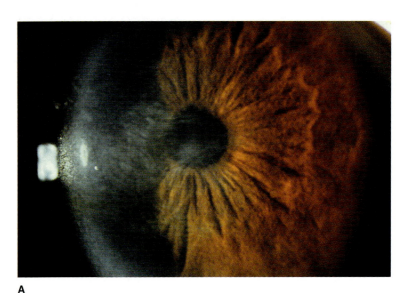

A

Figure 7-10 Interstitial keratitis A. *This patient with a history of congenital syphilis has old corneal stromal scarring. The clearer lines are old blood vessels. The scarring may be mid stromal or posterior stromal and there is often moderate corneal thinning. (Continued.)*

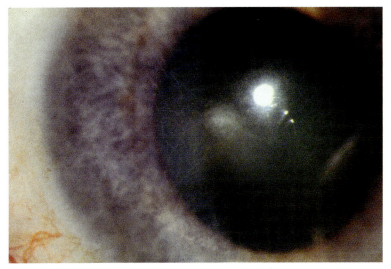

B

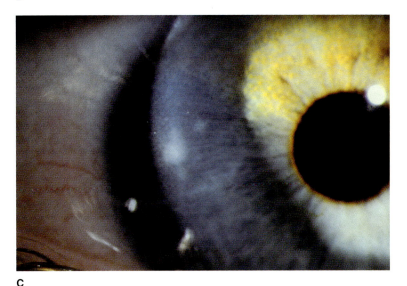

C

Figure 7-10 (cont.) Interstitial keratitis B. *Numerous corneal stromal "ghost" vessels are seen. The patient had a history of congenital syphilis.* **C.** *Nummular corneal infiltrates are present in this eye of a patient with Lyme disease. The patient was treated systemically for Lyme disease and the infiltrates responded to topical corticosteroids.*

SUBEPITHELIAL INFILTRATES

Subepithelial infiltrates are a common unilateral or bilateral keratopathy typically caused by viruses.

Etiology

- Adenovirus or Epstein-Barr virus infection
- Blepharitis, ocular rosacea
- Contact lens–induced reaction to preservatives in lens care solutions
- Thygeson's superficial punctate keratopathy
- Staphylococcal or chlamydial infections
- Lyme disease
- Epithelial corneal graft rejection in donor cornea (Krachmer's spots)

Symptoms

- Photophobia, foreign body sensation, redness, tearing, mild blurring of vision

Signs

- Few or multiple, unilateral or bilateral, granular, small, oval or circular, subepithelial opacities which may stain with rose bengal but stain poorly with fluorescein (Figure 7-11)

Differential Diagnosis

- Superficial punctate keratopathy: multiple punctate epithelial defects which stain well with fluorescein but not with rose bengal.

Treatment

- Treat underlying condition.
- Preservative-free artificial tear drops or gels q 2 to 6 h and lubricating ointment qhs or bid.
- Mild topical corticosteroid (e.g., loteprednol 0.2% or fluorometholone drops 0.1% qid) if vision is affected or symptoms are severe. May require a slow taper to prevent recurrence.

Prognosis

- Good, especially if underlying condition can be identified. When corticosteroids are used, they often must be tapered very slowly to prevent recurrence.

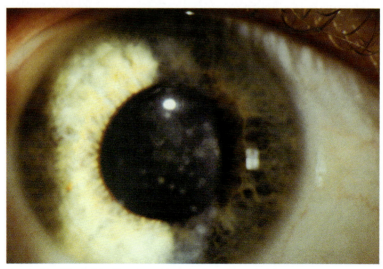

Figure 7-11 Subepithelial infiltrates after viral conjunctivitis *Multiple subepithelial infiltrates can be seen centrally in this eye several months after adenoviral keratoconjunctivitis causing glare, halos, and decreased vision.*

SUPERFICIAL PUNCTATE KERATOPATHY (PUNCTATE EPITHELIAL EROSIONS)

Superficial punctate keratopathy is a very common nonspecific finding seen in a wide variety of corneal disorders.

Etiology

Primarily Superior
- Subtarsal foreign body or concretions
- Vernal keratoconjunctivitis
- Superior limbic keratoconjunctivitis
- Trachoma
- Poorly fitting contact lens
- Floppy eyelid syndrome
- Trichiasis or distichiasis

Primarily Interpalpebral
- Keratoconjunctivitis sicca
- Neurotrophic keratopathy
- Exposure to ultraviolet light
- Contact lens–related (chemical toxicity, tight lens syndrome, overwear syndrome)

Primarily Inferior
- Rosacea, blepharitis
- Exposure keratopathy
- Lower eyelid margin lesions
- Toxicity from drops or chemical injury
- Entropion or ectropion
- Trichiasis or distichiasis
- Trauma, chemical injury
- Self inflicted, eye rubbing

Symptoms

- Foreign body sensation, tearing, and decreased of vision if central cornea is affected

Signs

- Multiple, tiny, pinpoint epithelial defects which stain well with fluorescein. They may be confluent if severe (Figures 7-12A,B).

Differential Diagnosis

- Subepithelial infiltrates: few or multiple, unilateral or bilateral, granular, small epithelial or subepithelial opacities which may stain with rose bengal but stain poorly with fluorescein

Treatment

- Treat underlying disorder.
- Discontinue contact lens wear and toxic medications.
- Preservative-free artificial tear drops or gels q 1 to 6 h and lubricating ointment qhs or bid depending on severity. Consider punctal occlusion.
- Topical antibiotic ointment (e.g., erythromycin or tetracycline) 2 to 4 times a day may be added.
- Avoid topical medications containing preservatives.

Prognosis

- Generally good, but depends on the underlying condition.

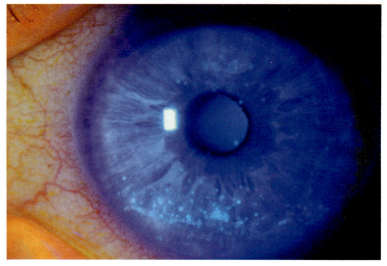

A

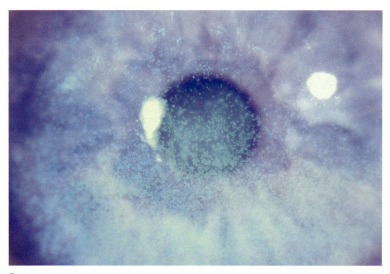

B

Figure 7-12 Superficial punctate keratopathy *A. Fluorescein dye and cobalt blue light reveal significant inferior corneal punctate staining. B. Fluorescein dye and cobalt blue light demonstrate severe central punctate staining. The staining is almost confluent inferiorly.*

THYGESON'S SUPERFICIAL PUNCTATE KERATOPATHY

Thygeson's superficial punctate keratopathy is an uncommon, usually bilateral, idiopathic condition that has a chronic course with exacerbations and remissions. It may resolve spontaneously after many years.

Etiology

- Unknown. Some physicians believe it is of viral origin.

Symptoms

- Photophobia, foreign body sensation, tearing, mildly decreased vision.

Signs

- Course, punctate or stellate, round to oval grayish-white clusters of epithelial lesions which usually occur centrally, are slightly elevated, and stain minimally with fluorescein (Figures 7-13A,B).
- The conjunctiva is not injected and the anterior chamber is quiet.

Treatment

- Artificial tear drops q 2 to 6 h and lubricating ointment qhs or bid depending on severity.
- Mild topical corticosteroid if vision is affected or symptoms are severe (e.g., loteprednol 0.2% or fluorometholone drops 0.1% qid). Corticosteroid drops can usually be tapered, but recurrence is common. A few patients may need long-term low-dose corticosteroids to remain asymptomatic.
- Therapeutic soft contact lenses may provide symptomatic relief if corticosteroid therapy fails or is contraindicated.
- Topical cyclosporine drops have been reported to help in certain patients.

Prognosis

- Good for significantly improved symptoms, but the condition is often chronic and recurrent.

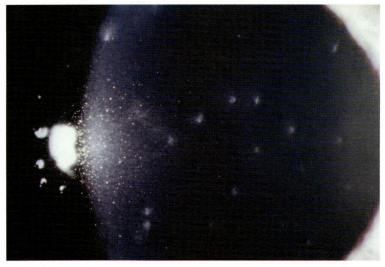

A

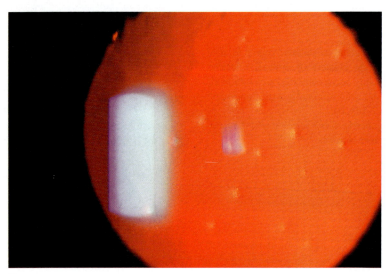

B

Figure 7-13   Thygeson's superficial punctate keratopathy   A. *Multiple, small epithelial lesions are present in the central cornea. They may stain minimally with fluorescein dye* **B.** *The same eye as in* **Figure 7-13A** *seen with retroillumination off the retina. Note the coarse, slightly stellate nature of the epithelial lesions.*

KERATOCONJUNCTIVITIS SICCA (DRY EYE SYNDROME)

Keratoconjunctivitis sicca refers to a dry eye syndrome which commonly causes chronic low-grade irritation of the eyes. It is primarily caused by aqueous tear deficiency. It is often exacerbated by blepharitis and meibomitis.

Etiology

- Sjögren's syndrome (primary or secondary)
- Drugs (e.g., antihistamines, β-blockers, atropine)
- Collagen vascular diseases (e.g., rheumatoid arthritis, systemic lupus erythematosus, polymyositis, etc.)
- Conjunctival scarring (e.g., ocular cicatricial pemphigoid, Stevens-Johnson syndrome, trachoma, chemical injuries)
- Lacrimal gland destruction (e.g., tumor, sarcoidosis, surgical removal, radiation)
- Vitamin A deficiency (xerophthalmia)
- Idiopathic (involutional)

Symptoms

- Burning, foreign-body sensation, dryness, itching, tired feeling, mucous discharge.
- Paradoxically, some patients complain of episodes of tearing which is likely reflex tearing from severe keratopathy.
- Symptoms tend to be worse at the end of the day, with prolonged reading, in dry or dusty environments, and during contact lens wear.

Signs

- Reduced or absent tear meniscus
- Interpalpebral staining of conjunctiva and cornea with fluorescein, rose bengal, or lissamine green (Figure 7-14A)
- Corneal filaments and mucous plaques
- May have corneal neovascularization, thinning, scarring, ulceration or perforation, especially when associated with collagen vascular diseases (Figures 7-14B,C)

Differential Diagnosis

- Other causes of superficial punctate keratopathy (see section on Superficial Punctate Keratopathy, above).

Diagnosis

- Keratoconjunctivitis sicca is a clinical diagnosis based on a combination of history, clinical signs, and ancillary tests.
- Abnormal Schirmer's test (<5 to 10 mm with anesthesia or <10 to 15 mm without anesthesia after 5 minutes).
- Reduced tear film break-up time (moderate: <10 seconds, severe: <5 seconds).
- Decreased tear turnover (e.g., decreased dye clearance).

Treatment

- Tear replacement: artificial tear drops q 1 to 6 h (e.g., minimally preserved tears in bottles when used qid or less, preservative-free tears in plastic vials when used greater than qid).
- Avoid aggravating factors (e.g., dry, dusty environment) and treat associated conditions (e.g., blepharitis, meibomitis).
- Tear ointment at bedtime or more frequent in severe cases.
- Punctal occlusion: collagen plugs (temporary), silicone plugs (reversible) (Figure 7-14D), or punctal cautery (permanent).
- Eye patch, moist chamber, or small lateral tarsorrhaphy can aid in tear preservation.
- Filaments can be removed mechanically with forceps. Acetylcysteine 10% drops (e.g., Mucomyst®) qid can help in filamentary keratopathy.
- Topical cyclosporine 0.02 to 0.5% drops may be of some benefit in certain patients.
- Work-up and treat underlying systemic disorders, especially collagen vascular conditions, if severe.

Prognosis

- Good for improvement in symptoms, but it depends on the underlying etiology. Most causes are chronic and require chronic therapy.

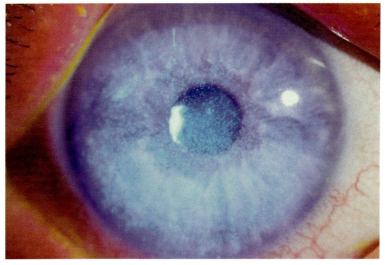

A

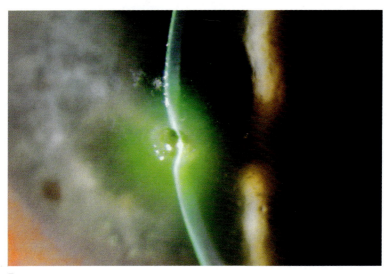

B

Figure 7-14 **Keratoconjunctivitis sicca** **A.** *Severe superficial punctate epitheliopathy is present centrally and inferiorly in this patient with severe dry eye syndrome. Inferiorly the keratopathy is confluent.* **B.** *A deep sterile corneal melt is present in this eye with severe dry eye syndrome. The slit-lamp beam reveals approximately 90% tissue loss. (Continued.)*

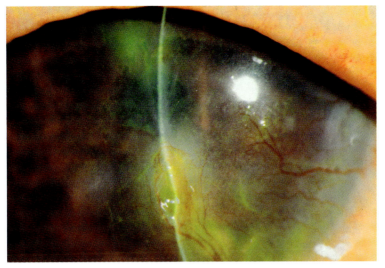

C

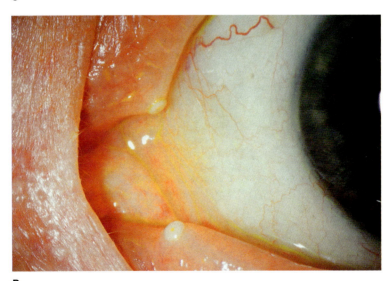

D

Figure 7-14 (cont.) Keratoconjunctivitis sicca C. *This eye developed a corneal perforation due to severe dry eye syndrome. It was treated with corneal tissue adhesive and sealed. Significant corneal thinning, scarring, and neovascularization remain.* **D.** *Silicone punctal plugs are present in the upper and lower tear drainage ducts of this eye with dry eye syndrome. The plugs prevent the tears from draining into the lacrimal system, thereby remaining in the eye longer to lubricate the ocular surface. They are most beneficial in patients with decreased tear production.*

FILAMENTARY KERATOPATHY

Filamentary keratopathy is a relatively common, unilateral or bilateral condition arising from aberrant healing of the epithelium. It can be caused by a variety of disorders.

Etiology

- Keratoconjunctivitis sicca
- Prolonged eye patching or ptosis
- Superior limbic keratoconjunctivitis
- Recurrent corneal erosions
- Neurotrophic/exposure keratopathy
- Diminished corneal sensation
- Essential blepharospasm
- Postoperative, near wound
- Midbrain strokes

Symptoms

- Foreign-body sensation, pain, redness, decreased vision

Signs

- Mucus threads containing desquamated epithelial cells that stain with fluorescein attached at one end to the corneal epithelium, conjunctival injection, punctate epithelial erosions, abnormal tear film (Figure 7-15)

Treatment

- Work-up and treat underlying disorder.
- Lubrication with preservative-free artificial tear drops q 1 to 6 h and ointment qhs. Punctal occlusion if dry.
- Debridement of filaments at their base using a pair of jeweler's forceps under topical anesthesia.
- Acetylcysteine 10% drops (e.g. Mucomyst®) qid.
- Bandage soft contact lens with topical antibiotic drops bid for a few weeks if symptoms are severe or if medications have failed, if not associated with significant dry eye.

Prognosis

- Good for improvement in symptoms, but prognosis depends on the underlying etiology. Most causes are chronic and require chronic therapy.

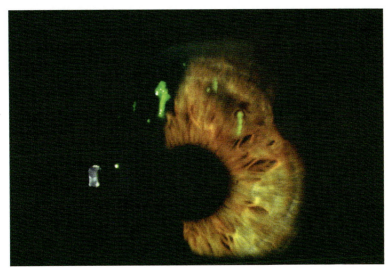

Figure 7-15   Filamentary keratopathy   *Several filaments (epithelial mucoid strands) which stain with fluorescein dye are present superiorly in this patient with dry eye syndrome.*

EXPOSURE KERATOPATHY

Exposure keratopathy is caused by drying of the ocular surface as a result of abnormal eyelid blinking or incomplete eyelid closure.

Etiology

- Facial nerve palsy
- Eyelid malpositions (e.g., ectropion or scarring after ptosis surgery or trauma)
- Nocturnal lagophthalmos
- Proptosis (e.g., dysthyroid eye disease)
- Eyelid coloboma
- After blepharoplasty or eyelid excision for tumors

Symptoms

- Irritation, burning, foreign-body sensation, tearing, epiphora, decreased vision
- May have a history of sleeping with eyes open

Signs

- Eyelid deformity or malposition can be noted (Figure 7-16).
- Incomplete blinking or closure of eyelids.
- Corneal desiccation with loss of normal luster, punctate epithelial erosions or epithelial defect affecting mainly the inferior interpalpebral region.
- In more severe cases, pannus, sterile ulceration, secondary infection, or rarely perforation can develop.

Treatment

- Correct underlying eyelid disorder.
- Lubrication with artificial tears/gels (more viscous preparations are preferred) q 1 to 4 h during the day and tear ointment or antibiotic ointment at night.
- Alternatively, artificial tear or antibiotic ointment qid can be used.
- Eyelid taping or patching at bedtime with ointments.
- Tarsorrhaphy or gold weight implant in the upper eyelid can be considered for more permanent treatment.

Prognosis

- Fair to good, depending on the underlying etiology. Worse if associated with decreased corneal sensation or a poor Bell's phenomenon.

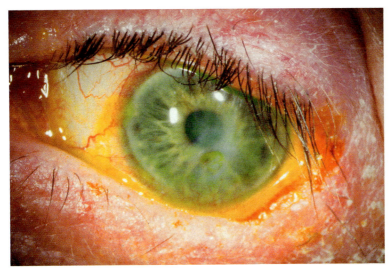

Figure 7-16 Exposure keratopathy *This patient has an inferior eyelid abnormality leading to poor eyelid coverage and exposure keratopathy. Corneal thinning and scarring from previous corneal ulceration can be noted inferocentrally.*

NEUROTROPHIC KERATOPATHY

Neurotrophic keratopathy occurs in eyes with diminished corneal sensation. It is usually acquired but can rarely be congenital.

Etiology

- Previous herpes zoster or simplex infection
- After ocular surgery (e.g., corneal transplantation, laser-assisted in-situ keratomileusis [LASIK])
- Radiation keratopathy
- Eye drops (e.g., anesthetic, timolol, non-steroidal anti-inflammatory agents)
- Chronic contact lens wear
- Section of the trigeminal nerve for tic douloureux
- Stroke
- Longstanding diabetes, especially after eye surgery
- Leprosy
- Familial dysautonomia (Riley-Day syndrome)

Symptoms

- Redness, tearing, burning, foreign-body sensation, decreased vision.

Signs

- Interpalpebral punctate epithelial erosions.
- Epithelial defects with built-up edges that are slow to heal and stain with fluorescein (Figure 7-17A).
- Secondary infection may occur.
- In severe cases, sterile ulceration, keratitis, iritis, and hypopyon can be seen (Figure 7-17B).
- Corneal perforation may occur in advanced cases.

Treatment

- The mainstay of treatment is lubrication with preservative-free artificial tears/gels (more viscous preparations are preferred) q 1 to 4 h during the day and tear ointment or antibiotic ointment at night.
- Alternatively, artificial tear ointment or antibiotic ointment q 1 to 6 h can be substituted.
- In cases with ulceration, patching, tarsorrhaphy, botulinum toxin injection to induce ptosis, amniotic membrane graft, or conjunctival flap can be employed.

Prognosis

- Fair, depending on underlying etiology. The goal is to prevent secondary complications as the nerves may not regenerate a great deal.

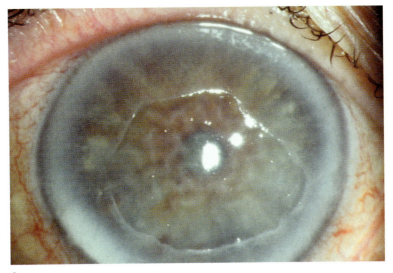

A

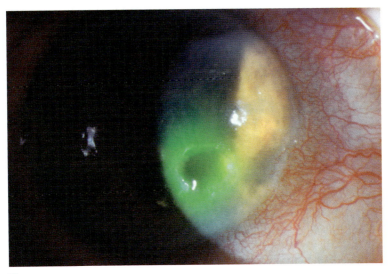

B

Figure 7-17 Neurotrophic keratopathy A. *A large central corneal epithelial defect is present. The thickened rolled-up edges are classic signs of neurotrophic keratopathy. There is underlying corneal edema.* **Neurotrophic corneal melt B.** *Two months after uncomplicated temporal clear corneal cataract extraction with phacoemulsification, a small sterile corneal melt developed at the cataract wound and a large deep sterile melt developed inferonasally. The patient had been using ketorolac for several weeks for mild corneal edema. The limbal ulcer resolved upon discontinuation of the ketorolac and the addition of lubricants. The larger ulcer responded well to cyanoacrylate corneal glue.*

RECURRENT CORNEAL EROSION

Recurrent corneal erosion typically occurs in eyes that have previously sustained acute, sharp abrasion (e.g., from a fingernail, tree branch, or paper edge injury) to the cornea and in eyes with corneal dystrophies.

Etiology and Pathophysiology

- Previous traumatic corneal abrasion.
- Corneal dystrophy (e.g., anterior basement membrane [ABM], Meesmann's, Reis-Bücklers', lattice, granular dystrophies), may have a family history.
- Diabetes mellitus.
- Disturbance to Bowman's layer, resulting in defective hemidesmosomal attachment of the epithelium to the basement membrane. The loosely attached epithelium is easily eroded and this perpetuates the disturbance and is responsible for the recurrent nature of the disorder.

Symptoms

- Recurrent attacks of acute, sharp pain typically during sleep or upon awakening
- History of superficial corneal injury
- Tearing, photophobia, mild to severe blurring of vision

Signs

- Localized epithelial irregularities with negative fluorescein staining (Figures 7-18A,B).
- Epithelial defect may sometimes be seen during acute stages.
- Dots, microcysts, and fingerprint patterns of ABM dystrophy may best be seen with retro-illumination. Other corneal dystrophies can be seen on slit-lamp examination, so check both eyes.

Treatment

- Artificial tear drops q 2 to 6 h and lubricating ointment qhs or lubricating ointment q 2 to 6 h.
- Topical antibiotic ointment (e.g., erythromycin or tetracycline) 2 to 4 times a day until the epithelial defect has healed.
- Cycloplegics (scopolamine 0.25% or cyclopentolate 1% tid) if iritis is present.
- Consider a pressure patch for 24 hours during acute stages.
- Once healing is complete: artificial tear drops qid and ointment qhs or sodium chloride 5% drops qid and ointment qhs for at least 3 months.

If epithelium is grossly loose, recurrence is frequent, or when medical therapy fails, the following measures can be considered:

- Epithelial debridement.
- Anterior stromal micropuncture for small areas of erosions outside the visual axis (Figures 7-18C,D).
- Diamond burr polishing of Bowman's membrane for larger areas of erosions.
- Excimer laser phototherapeutic keratectomy (PTK) for larger areas of erosions.
- Bandage soft contact lens for 3 months.

Prognosis

- Very good to excellent with proper management. Recurrences can occur even with surgical treatment, but surgery can be repeated.

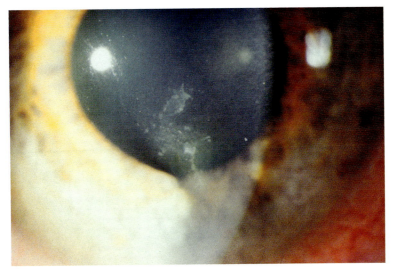

A

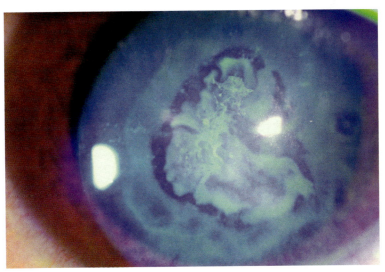

B

Figure 7-18   Recurrent erosion syndrome   *A. An area of loose, gray, thickened epithelium is seen in this eye with a healing recurrent erosion. In eyes with mild erosions, the slit-lamp examination may be essentially normal several hours after an erosion. One must look carefully for epithelial irregularities. B. After fluorescein stain using a cobalt blue light, a large area of loose epithelium is quite apparent. Areas of negative staining indicate elevated, thickened epithelium. Centrally, mild fluorescein staining is present where the epithelial defect has almost completely healed. (Continued.)*

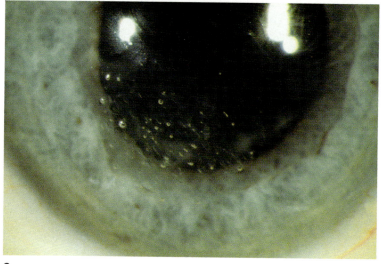

C

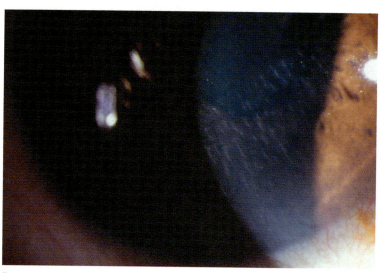

D

Figure 7-18 (cont.)   Recurrent erosion syndrome   **C.** *This photograph was taken immediately after anterior stromal micropuncture was performed. Under slit-lamp illumination, approximately 150 small punctures into the anterior 20% of the cornea were performed with a 25 gauge needle in the area of recurrent erosion. Numerous tiny air bubbles under the epithelium are present.* **D.** *Three months after anterior stromal micropuncture for recurrent erosion syndrome, multiple tiny linear scars can be seen. Ideally, this procedure is performed outside of the visual axis, as occasionally these scars can affect vision.*

BULLOUS KERATOPATHY

Bullous keratopathy is a fairly common condition due to endothelial decompensation and is characterized by corneal edema.

Etiology

- Postoperative endothelial damage (e.g., aphakic or pseudophakic bullous keratopathy) (Figures 7-19A,B)
- Endothelial dystrophy (e.g., Fuchs', posterior polymorphous, congenital hereditary)
- Corneal graft failure
- Blunt or penetrating anterior segment trauma (e.g., forceps delivery, ocular trauma)
- Iridocorneal endothelial syndrome (e.g., Chandler's syndrome)
- Acute angle closure glaucoma
- Brown-McLean syndrome: peripheral corneal edema often associated with aphakia (Figure 7-19C)

Symptoms

- Decreased vision, redness, tearing, foreign-body sensation, pain, photophobia.

Signs

- Corneal stromal and epithelial edema, superficial vesicles or bullae, epithelial defects from ruptured bullae, Descemet's folds, cornea guttata
- In longstanding cases, may have neovascularization, subepithelial or stromal scarring

Diagnosis

- Pachymetry shows an increase in corneal thickness.
- Specular microscopy demonstrates decreased endothelial cell density.

Treatment

- Topical sodium chloride 5% drops qid and ointment qhs to reduce epithelial edema.
- Topical antibiotic ointment qid for ruptured bullae. Patching or bandage soft contact lenses can also be considered.
- Cycloplegics (scopolamine 0.25% or cyclopentolate 1% tid) if iritis is present.
- Blow warm air over the cornea for 10 minutes in the morning to reduce corneal edema.
- Corneal transplant for visual rehabilitation if medical treatment fails. Old style (closed loop and iris-fixated) intraocular lenses should be removed.
- For symptomatic relief in a painful eye with poor visual potential, consider anterior stromal micropuncture, conjunctival flap or amniotic membrane transplant.
- Control glaucoma and any associated iritis.

Prognosis

- Mild cases may retain reasonable vision and good comfort for years, but the endothelial cell loss is usually progressive. Success rate is generally good with corneal transplantation.

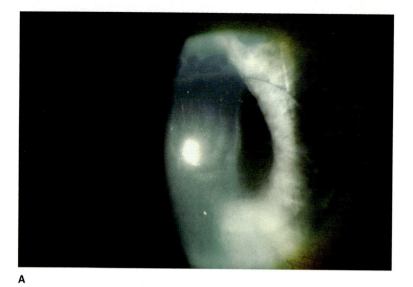

A

B

Figure 7-19   Bullous keratopathy   A. *This eye has significant corneal edema, greater inferiorly than superiorly. There is a closed loop, Leiske anterior chamber intraocular lens implant. Closed loop anterior chamber intraocular lens implants were strongly associated with causing bullous keratopathy, often requiring corneal transplantation to achieve better vision. During corneal transplantation, these lenses are removed.* **B.** *Significant diffuse corneal stromal edema can be seen in this eye with an open loop anterior chamber intraocular lens implant. (Continued.)*

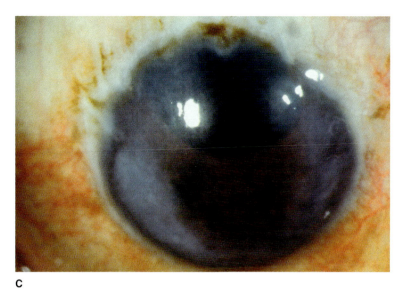

C

Figure 7-19 (cont.)   Brown-McLean syndrome   C. *Pronounced peripheral corneal edema is present in this aphakic eye. The chronic corneal edema has caused subepithelial fibrosis. The vision remains rather good as the central cornea is relatively clear.*

ACQUIRED IMMUNE DEFICIENCY SYNDROME (AIDS)

AIDS is a condition characterized by the presence of opportunistic infections, Kaposi's sarcoma, and/or lymphoma in an immunocompromised patient infected with the human immunodeficiency virus.

Etiology

- Human immunodeficiency virus (HIV)

Symptoms

- May be asymptomatic; other symptoms depend on the specific problem.

Eye Signs

- Nonspecific follicular conjunctivitis, punctate epithelial keratitis, conjunctival microangiopathy, episcleritis, iritis may occur (Figure 7-20A)
- Herpes zoster ophthalmicus
- Molluscum contagiosum: may have extensive lesions with minimal conjunctivitis.
- Kaposi's sarcoma of eyelid or conjunctiva: reddish-purple subepidermal or subepithelial nodule. The subconjunctival lesion may be mistaken for a subconjunctival hemorrhage (Figure 7-20B).
- Microsporidial keratitis: chronic superficial punctate keratitis which does not respond to conventional treatment. Diagnosed by corneal scraping for Giemsa stain. Treatment is with topical fumagillin and oral itraconazole or albendazole. Improves as the immune status improves.
- Corneal endothelial deposits associated with cytomegalovirus (CMV) and HIV medications (Figure 7-20C)
- Fungal, herpes simplex, or cytomegalovirus keratitis may also be seen
- Retinal microangiopathy, CMV or *Candida* retinitis, *Pneumocystis carinii* or cryptococcal choroiditis, toxoplasma retinochoroiditis, ocular large cell lymphoma
- Syphilis
- Cranial nerve palsies, optic neuropathy

Diagnosis

- Enzyme-linked immunosorbent assay (ELISA) for serum HIV antibody
- Western blot test to confirm diagnosis

Treatment

- Systemic treatment by an internist or infectious disease specialist.
- Opportunistic infections are treated accordingly with antimicrobial medications.
- Kaposi's sarcoma: local irradiation, excision, cryotherapy, and/or systemic chemotherapy.

Prognosis

- Fair to poor, depending on the severity of the HIV disease.

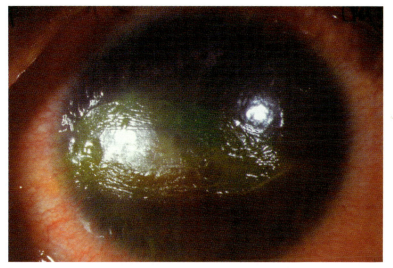

A

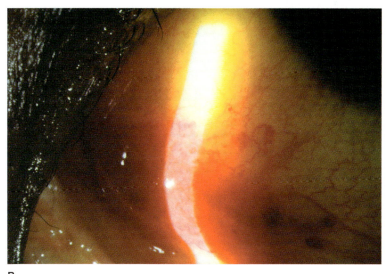

B

Figure 7-20 Acquired immune deficiency syndrome A. *Severe persistent conjunctivitis has caused a chronic keratitis and dry eye state. There is significant corneal neovascularization, especially inferiorly. The central cornea is keratinized from chronic surface disease.* **B.** *This subconjunctival vascular mass is a Kaposi's sarcoma. It may be mistakenly thought to be a subconjunctival hemorrhage, but it does not resolve over a few weeks. (Continued.)*

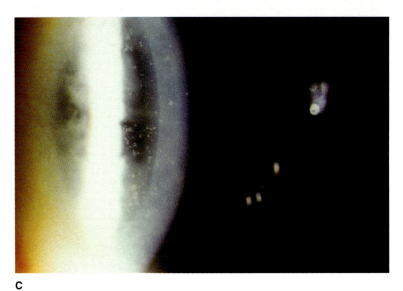

C

Figure 7-20 (cont.)   Acquired immune deficiency syndrome   C. *Multiple small, gray or pigmented endothelial deposits can be seen in patients with HIV disease. They are more prominent in the corneal periphery. They do not appear to directly affect vision. These deposits may be seen in patients with or without cytomegalovirus retinitis.*

CONTACT LENS COMPLICATIONS

TOXIC/ALLERGIC CONJUNCTIVITIS

Etiology

A hypersensitivity or toxic reaction usually caused by preservatives (e.g., thimerosal or chlorhexidine) in the contact lens solution.

Symptoms

Burning, itching, redness soon after lens insertion.

Signs

Conjunctival injection, follicular conjunctivitis, superficial punctate keratopathy.

Treatment

Lubrication with preservative-free artificial tears. Avoid solutions containing preservatives. Switch to a hydrogen peroxide system. Consider daily wear disposable lenses.

GIANT PAPILLARY CONJUNCTIVITIS

Etiology

A hypersensitivity reaction to protein build-up in contact lenses, especially with soft lenses and poor lens hygiene.

Symptoms

Itching, mucus discharge, burning, reduced lens tolerance.

Signs

Moderate- to giant-sized papillae on the upper tarsal conjunctiva, deposits may be seen on contact lens (Figures 7-21A,B). Contact lens may be high riding.

Treatment

Optimize lens hygiene and lens fitting. Increase frequency of enzyme deproteinization. Reduce duration of lens wear. Consider switching to frequent replacement/ daily disposable or rigid gas-permeable lenses. Topical lubrication and mast cell stabilizer (e.g., olopatadine bid or cromolyn qid).

CONTACT LENS KERATOPATHY (CONTACT LENS–ASSOCIATED SUPERIOR LIMBIC KERATOCONJUNCTIVITIS)

Etiology

Usually related to contact lens preservative hypersensitivity or toxicity or overwear.

Symptoms

Burning, itching, redness, reduced lens tolerance, occasionally decreased vision.

Signs

Superior conjunctival injection, superficial punctate keratitis, subepithelial infiltrates and haze. May have a superior corneal epitheliopathy (FIGURES 7-21c,d).

Treatment

Avoid solutions containing preservatives. Lubricate with preservative-free artificial tears. Switch to a hydrogen peroxide system. Consider switching to frequent replacement/daily disposable or rigid gas-permeable lenses.

CONTACT LENS OVERWEAR SYNDROME

Etiology

Chronic, long periods or extended wear of soft lenses.

Symptoms

Redness, foreign-body sensation, tearing, burning, blurred vision.

Signs

Diffuse conjunctival injection, epithelial edema, punctate epithelial erosions, mild iritis. Superficial or deep corneal neovascularization may be seen in chronic cases.

Treatment

Lubricate with artificial tears. Discontinue extended wear and switch to daily wear. Reduce daily wearing time. Refit with more gas-permeable, looser lenses.

TIGHT LENS SYNDROME

Etiology

Acute, tight fitting of a soft lens or rarely a rigid lens. Overnight wear of a daily lens. Acute hypoxia.

Symptoms

Irritation, redness, pain, blurred vision a few hours after lens insertion. Patients often have difficulty removing lenses.

Signs

Absence of lens movement on blinking, imprint of lens on conjunctiva after soft lens removal (or cornea after rigid lens removal) (Figure 7-21E), corneal epithelial and anterior stromal edema, punctate keratopathy, iritis, and sterile hypopyon.

Treatment

Discontinue contact lens wear. Lubricate with artificial tears. Consider cycloplegic drops. Refit with a daily wear, flatter, looser lens.

CORNEAL WARPAGE

Etiology

Typically due to prolonged wear of imperme-able (polymethylmethacrylate) hard lenses, but can be seen with rigid gas-permeable lenses and even soft lenses.

Symptoms

Spectacle blur.

Signs

Moderate to severe irregular astigmatism on ker-atometry and computerized corneal topography.

Treatment

Discontinue lens wear and allow corneal curva-ture to return to normal, which may take months. Once normalized, refit with a rigid gas-permeable lens or soft lens and monitor for stability.

CORNEAL NEOVASCULARIZATION

Etiology

Extended wear of soft lenses or chronic over-wear of tight, low-oxygen permeable lenses.

Symptoms

May be asymptomatic.

Signs

Peripheral, superficial, and occasionally stromal, neovascularization usually affecting the superior limbus, but may occur 360 degrees. May be ac-companied by lipid infiltrates.

Treatment

Discontinue contact lens wear. Consider topical corticosteroids in severe cases. Refit with daily wear disposable lenses or rigid gas-permeable lenses.

STERILE KERATITIS

Etiology

May be related to allergic conjunctivitis, superior limbic keratoconjunctivitis, overwear or tight-lens syndrome, reaction to lens care preservatives.

Symptoms

May be asymptomatic or have mild irritation.

Signs

Single or multiple, small, peripheral, epithelial or subepithelial opacities (Figure 7-21F). Occasionally, a sterile anterior stromal infiltrate or haze may be seen. It is important to distinguish it from an early microbial keratitis.

Treatment

Discontinue lens wear. Broad-spectrum antibiotic drops qid. Judicious use of topical corticosteroid qid once infection has been ruled out. Follow-up patient in 1 to 2 days.

MICROBIAL KERATITIS

Etiology

Bacterial, fungal, *Acanthamoeba* corneal infection.

Symptoms

Pain, irritation, redness, tearing, discharge, photophobia, blurred vision. May have a history of extended wear or topical corticosteroid usage for contact lens–related problem.

Signs

Conjunctival injection, corneal infiltrate, corneal ulcer, iritis, hypopyon.

Treatment

See Bacterial Keratitis at the beginning of this chapter.

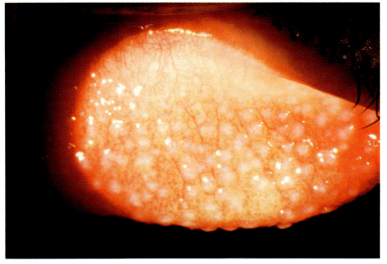

A

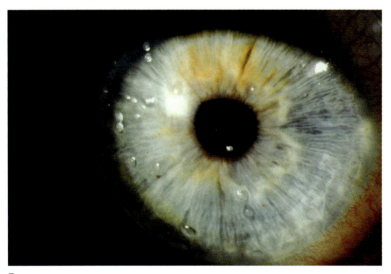

B

Figure 7-21 Contact lens complication   **A.** *Severe giant papillary conjunctivitis is present upon eversion of the upper eyelid in this patient who never enzymed his soft contact lenses and replaced them once a year.* **B.** *This soft contact lens is covered with thick, elevated protein deposit globules. The lens needs to be cleaned, enzymed, and disinfected. The patient needs to be instructed in proper lens care including more frequent enzyming and/or more frequent replacement. (Continued.)*

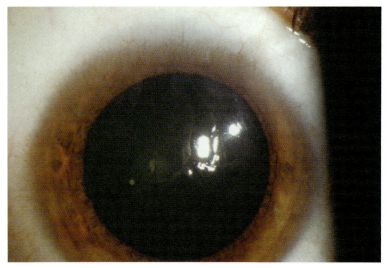

C

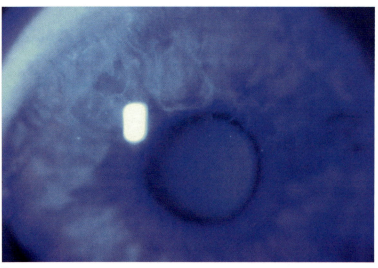

D

Figure 7-21 (cont.)   Contact lens complication   C. *This long-time soft contact lens wearer noted decreased vision. Tongues of irregular epithelium emanating from the superior limbus are apparent. Chronic irritation from contact lens wear can cause damage to the limbal stem cells resulting in abnormal epithelial cell production and irregular astigmatism.* **D.** *Fluorescein staining with a cobalt blue light highlights the irregular epithelium in a patient with a contact lens–induced limbal stem cell abnormality. (Continued.)*

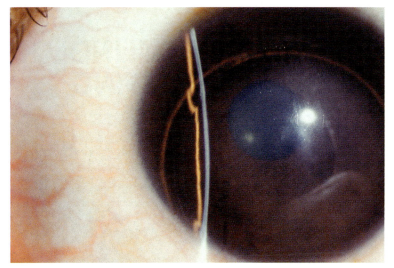

E

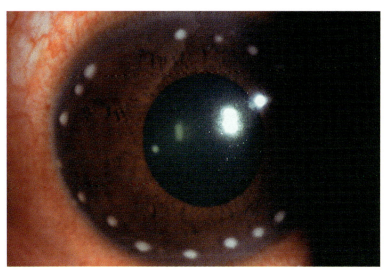

F

Figure 7-21 (cont.)   Contact lens complication   E. *A recently fit rigid gas-permeable contact lens was too tight. It had just been removed and the indentation of the "sucked-on" lens can still be seen in the cornea. The cornea needs to return to normal before the contact lens can be refit.* **F.** *Multiple peripheral corneal infiltrates are seen in this soft contact lens wearer's eye. It was thought to be due to a toxic reaction to preservatives in the contact lens cleaning solution.*

Chapter 8

SYSTEMIC AND IMMUNOLOGIC CONDITIONS AFFECTING THE CORNEA

WILSON'S DISEASE (HEPATOLENTICULAR DEGENERATION)

Wilson's disease is a rare condition resulting in abnormal copper deposition throughout the body.

Etiology and Epidemiology

- Autosomal recessive condition caused by a deficiency of the enzyme ceruloplasmin
- Onset under age 40 years

Symptoms

- Usually no ocular symptoms
- May experience cirrhosis, renal disease, or neurologic dysfunction (typically motor disorders)

Ocular Signs

- Kayser-Fleischer ring: green-brown band of copper deposition in the peripheral zone of Descemet's membrane (Figure 8-1; see also Figure 6-8). This ring usually begins in the vertical meridians and may be seen earliest with gonioscopy. A Kayser-Fleischer ring may be the presenting sign of the disease.
- Cataract is found in less than 10% of cases. A disc-shaped, central, polychromatic opacity with peripheral radiations can be seen (sunflower cataract).

Differential Diagnosis

- Other causes of a Kayser-Fleischer ring: primary biliary cirrhosis, chronic active hepatitis, multiple myeloma
- Chalchosis: corneal copper deposition from an intraocular copper foreign body

Diagnosis

- Slit-lamp or gonioscopic examination
- Serum copper and ceruloplasmin levels, urine copper level

Treatment

- Treatment by an internist and/or neurologist with copper chelating agents such as D-penicillamine or tetrathiomolybdate.

Prognosis

- Good with early recognition and treatment. Treatment may be followed by resolution of the Kayser-Fleischer ring.

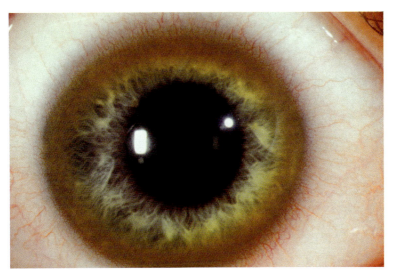

Figure 8-1   Wilson's disease   *A prominent Kayser-Fleischer ring can be seen. Brown copper pigment deposition is very apparent in the corneal periphery in this 18-year-old woman with Wilson's disease. The deposits are at the level of Descemet's membrane and deep stroma. In mild cases, the copper pigment is seen earliest using gonioscopy. See also **Figure 6-8**.*

VITAMIN A DEFICIENCY

Vitamin A deficiency is a rare, potentially blinding disorder usually affecting the malnourished that is common in areas where polished rice is the main source of food.

Etiology

- Dietary deficiency of vitamin A, typically from chronic malnutrition
- Celiac diseases, biliary obstruction, cystic fibrosis, pancreatic or intestinal (e.g., gastric stapling) surgery, which impairs absorption of vitamin A

Symptoms

- Night blindness is the earliest symptom, dry eye, foreign body sensation, gradual loss of vision in severe cases

Signs

- Xerosis of cornea and conjunctiva
- Keratinization of conjunctiva (Bitot's spot: superficial, triangular, silvery-gray, foamy, keratinized patch on the interpalpebral bulbar conjunctiva)
- Sterile corneal ulcers and melts (keratomalacia) which may lead to scarring or perforation (Figure 8-2).

Differential Diagnosis

- Keratoconjunctivitis sicca

Diagnosis

- Serum vitamin A level.
- Consider impression cytology of the conjunctiva (demonstrates decreased goblet cell density) and electroretinogram.

Treatment

- Systemic vitamin A orally or intramuscularly and repeated 1 month later.
- Frequent preservative-free artificial tear drops or ointment to lubricate ocular surface.
- Treat malnutrition.
- Corneal transplantation for scars or perforation. Consider a keratoprosthesis for bilateral severe scarring.

Prognosis

- Very good if diagnosed and treated before significant corneal ulceration has occurred. Fair to poor if significant corneal damage is present.

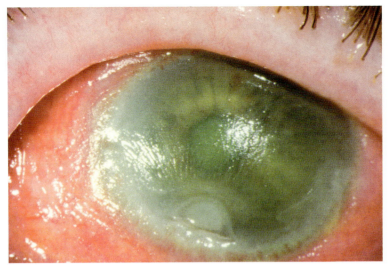

Figure 8-2 Vitamin A deficiency *This malnourished patient had severe xerosis of the cornea and conjunctiva. There was a deep sterile corneal melt near the limbus from the 6 to 7 o'clock positions. The xerosis and melt resolved over a week with systemic vitamin A therapy.*

CYSTINOSIS

Cystinosis is a rare disorder resulting in accumulation of cystine in the body.

Etiology and Epidemiology

- Autosomal recessive disorder.
- Results in deposits of the amino acid cystine in the conjunctiva, corneal stroma, iris, lens, and retina depending on severity.

Three Main Forms
- Infantile: associated with dwarfism and progressive kidney dysfunction. Poor prognosis without a renal transplant.
- Adolescent (intermediate): kidneys may be involved, but retina normal.
- Adult: minimal to no kidney disease, cystine deposits limited to anterior segment.

Symptoms

- Irritation, foreign body sensation, pain, occasionally decreased vision

Signs

- Myriad tiny, glistening crystals in the corneal stroma, conjunctiva, iris, lens, and retina, depending on the severity of the disease (Figures 8-3A,B).
- May have superficial punctate keratopathy, filaments, and recurrent erosions.
- There is growth retardation, renal failure, hepatosplenomegaly, and hypothyroidism.

Differential Diagnosis

- See Crystalline Keratopathy in Chapter 6, page 137.

Treatment

- Lubrication for ocular surface disease.
- Cysteamine eye drops have been reported to be useful.
- Rarely, a corneal transplant is required.

Prognosis

- Poor for the infantile form, good for the intermediate and adult forms.

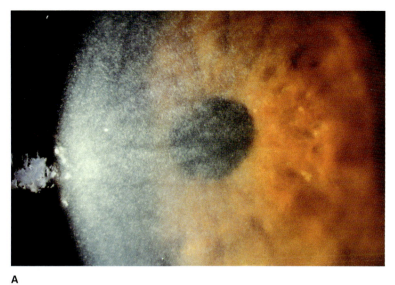

A

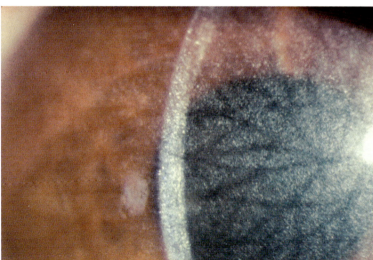

B

Figure 8-3   Cystinosis   A. *Confluent full-thickness tiny refractile corneal deposits are seen. These opacities are cystine crystals. Generally, the deposits do not affect vision; however if severe, they can cause significant visual symptoms.* **B.** *Slit-lamp beam view of the eye with cystinosis seen in Figure 8-3A. Note the full-thickness distribution of the crystals.*

MUCOPOLYSACCHARIDOSES AND LIPIDOSES

A group of inherited systemic metabolic disorders resulting in abnormal accumulation of material in the body.

Etiology and Epidemiology

Mucopolysaccharidoses Lysosomal storage diseases including Hurler, Scheie, Hunter, Sanfilippo, Morquio, Maroteaux-Lamy and Sly syndromes. All are autosomal recessive except Hunter syndrome which is X-linked recessive.

Lipidoses Numerous disorders of lipid metabolism, including Fabry's disease. All lipidoses are autosomal recessive except Fabry's disease which is X-linked recessive.

Ocular Signs

Mucopolysaccharidoses All may have optic nerve, retinal, and CNS abnormalities. All have progressive corneal clouding except Hunter and Sanfilippo (Figure 8-4).

Lipidoses All may have macular cherry-red spots and optic atrophy. Bilateral, symmetrical, brownish corneal epithelial deposits arranged in a vortex fashion from a point below the pupil and swirling outward but sparing the limbus (cornea verticillata) is seen in males with Fabry's disease and female carriers. Conjunctival aneurysms, lens opacities, papilledema, optic atrophy, and macular and retinal edema are also seen in Fabry's disease.

Treatment

- Severe corneal opacity may require a corneal transplant. No ocular treatment is required for cornea verticillata.
- Follow-up with a pediatrician or pediatric endocrinologist.

Prognosis

- Poor to good depending on the specific metabolic disorder.

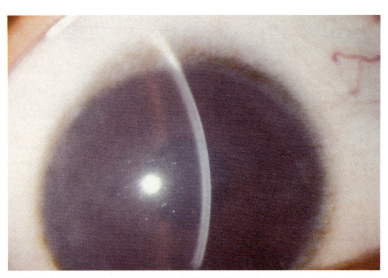

Figure 8-4 Maroteaux-Lamy syndrome *Diffuse full-thickness corneal haze can be seen in this child with Maroteaux-Lamy syndrome.*

COLLAGEN VASCULAR DISEASES

Collagen vascular diseases can cause a wide variety of ocular abnormalities, the most important of which is scleritis.

Etiology

- Rheumatoid arthritis (most common)
- Wegener's granulomatosis (often causes a necrotizing scleritis)
- Polyarteritis nodosa
- Relapsing polychondritis
- Systemic lupus erythematosus (SLE)

Symptoms

- Range from minimal to significant pain, redness, discharge, decreased vision.

Signs

- Corneal findings include keratoconjunctivitis sicca, stromal keratitis, corneal stromal infiltrates or ulceration, typically peripheral but may be central. The peripheral corneal ulceration may occur with or without inflammation. The ulceration can be similar to Mooren's ulcer in that it can extend circumferentially and centrally. However, unlike Mooren's ulcer, the sclera is commonly involved. Corneal perforation may occur (Figures 8-5A,B,C).
- Other findings include episcleritis, scleritis (necrotizing with or without inflammation) and sclerokeratitis (Figure 8-5D). Healed episodes of scleritis can lead to scleral thinning and uveal show (Figure 8-5E).
- The corneal changes in SLE are often unremarkable.

Differential Diagnosis

- Mooren's ulcer: no underlying systemic disease
- Infectious infiltrate or ulcer: pain, iritis, more purulent discharge, cultures positive

Treatment

- Artificial tear drops, gels, and ointment, and punctal occlusion are used for keratoconjunctivitis sicca. Topical corticosteroids are helpful in stromal keratitis but should generally be avoided in corneal and scleral ulcers.
- Oral nonsteroidal anti-inflammatory agents and/or corticosteroids are used for peripheral ulcerative keratitis and scleritis. Topical treatment is aimed at reepithelialization and prevention of secondary infection (e.g., artificial tear and antibiotic ointment qid, punctal occlusion, lateral tarsorrhaphy).
- Stronger immunosuppressive agents (e.g., cyclophosphamide, methotrexate) may be required, especially for scleritis or corneal stromal inflammation.
- Resection of inflamed conjunctiva adjacent to a peripheral corneal ulcer may be helpful. Cyanoacrylate tissue glue can be used for small perforations. Larger perforations will require corneal patch grafts.

Prognosis

- Fair to good depending on the aggressiveness and response of the underlying systemic disease.

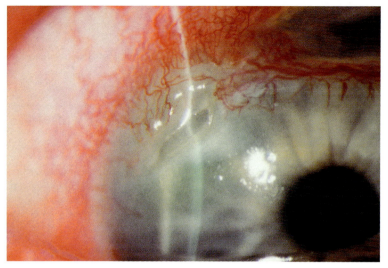

A

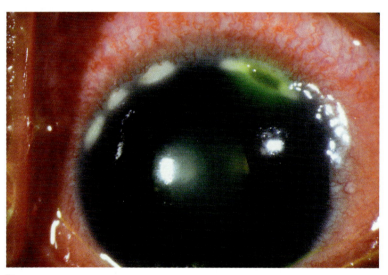

B

Figure 8-5   Rheumatoid arthritis   A. *Slit-lamp beam view of a patient with rheumatoid arthritis demonstrates a peripheral corneal melt with severe ulceration. There is approximately 90% tissue loss. There is moderate corneal neovascularization peripherally and superiorly. Note the area of clear cornea superiorly; it is an additional large area of corneal melting.* **B.** *This patient with rheumatoid arthritis has three separate peripheral corneal infiltrates from the 9 to 11 o'clock positions. There is an additional, larger peripheral infiltrate with corneal melting from the 12 to 2 o'clock positions. The infiltrates are most likely sterile, inflammatory infiltrates. (Continued.)*

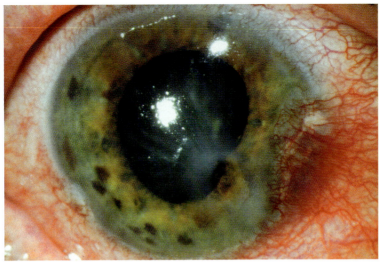

C

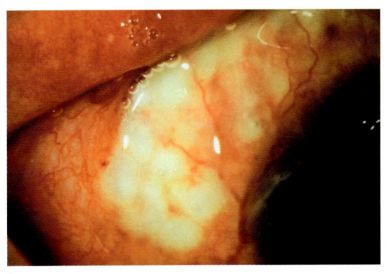

D

Figure 8-5 (cont.)   Rheumatoid arthritis   C. *This eye has a large sterile corneal melt leading to perforation in the midperiphery at the 5 o'clock position. The radiating stromal folds suggest a perforation. Peripheral corneal neovascularization and scarring from the 3 to 4 o'clock positions indicates previous corneal inflammation in that area.* **Wegener's granulomatosis   D.** *This patient with a necrotizing scleritis and peripheral corneal melt had no known medical problems. Emergent systemic work-up revealed Wegener's granulomatosis. She was treated aggressively with systemic corticosteroids and cyclophosphamide and her scleritis resolved. Appropriate diagnosis and treatment of Wegener's granulomatosis can be life-saving. (Continued.)*

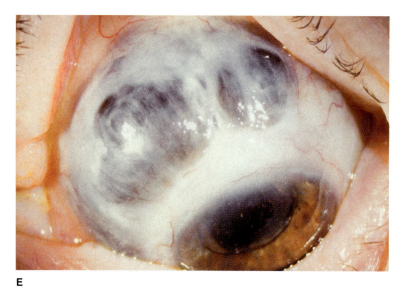

E

Figure 8-5 (cont.)   Rheumatoid arthritis   E. *This eye had previous, asymptomatic scleral inflammation (scleritis) with progressive loss of scleral tissue. The sclera has become so thin that the brown uveal tissue can be seen. This condition is termed scleromalacia perforans.*

OCULAR CICATRICIAL PEMPHIGOID

Cicatricial pemphigoid is an uncommon, chronic cicatrizing mucocutaneous disorder. Many patients also have lesions of the oral mucosa. The skin lesions are less common. Bilateral conjunctival involvement occurs in the majority of cases, and in some it may be the only manifestation of the disease.

Etiology and Epidemiology

- Idiopathic type II hypersensitivity reaction caused by anti-basement membrane antibodies
- Primarily female patients over 60 years of age
- Has been associated with numerous topical drugs (e.g., pilocarpine, timolol, idoxuridine)

Symptoms

- Chronic remitting and relapsing course, ocular redness, irritation, foreign-body sensation, decreased vision, generally progressive
- Oral ulcerations

Signs

- Bilateral, often asymmetric, conjunctival inflammation, fine subepithelial fibrosis of conjunctiva with shrinkage and obliteration of the inferior fornix, often with progressive symblepharon formation (Figures 8-6A,B).
- Trichiasis and distichiasis may lead to corneal pannus, scarring, thinning, ulceration, and occasionally perforation.
- Punctate epithelial erosions, poor tear film, dry eye, blepharoconjunctivitis.
- Corneal pannus or keratinization and fusion between the upper and lower eyelids at the outer canthus (Figure 8-6C).
- Corneal ulceration and vascularization which may be complicated by infection, persistent epithelial defects, exposure, and perforation.
- Mucous membrane vesicles and ulcerations (oral cavity, nose, anus).

Differential Diagnosis

- Stevens-johnson syndrome: acute onset, precipitated by drug or infection, generally does not run a remitting and relapsing course
- Chemical injury: acute onset, diagnosis is obvious from history

Diagnosis

- Pull down the lower eyelids while asking patient to look up to observe for inferior forniceal foreshortening and inferior symblepharon.
- Look for lesions in oral cavity and skin.
- Conjunctival biopsy to look for subepithelial bullae and subepithelial fibrosis, and for immunofluorescent identification of antigen-antibody complexes in the conjunctival basement membranes.

Treatment

- Artificial tear drops or ointments (e.g., q 2 to 6 h or ointment 2 to 4 times per day). Punctal occlusion for severe cases with either punctal plugs or punctal cautery.
- Treat any associated blepharitis with eyelid hygiene, topical antibiotic ointment, and oral tetracycline, doxycycline, or erythromycin. Treat trichiasis with epilation, electrolysis, and cryotherapy as needed.
- Topical corticosteroids (e.g., prednisolone 1%, dexamethasone 0.1%, or loteprednol 0.5% qid) for active conjunctival inflammation.
- Oral dapsone can be used alone or can complement other systemic treatment. Dapsone should be avoided in patients who have glucose-6-phosphate dehydrogenase (G6PD) deficiency.
- Systemic corticosteroid or immunosuppressives (e.g., cyclophosphamide, methotrexate, azathioprine) for treatment of active systemic and ocular disease.

- Surgical procedures should be planned carefully. Eyelid deformities can be reconstructed. Forniceal shortening may be corrected by mucous membrane or amniotic membrane grafts. Surgery may trigger inflammation.
- Limbal stem cell graft and corneal graft have a high failure rate. Keratoprosthesis can be considered if the eye has good visual potential and the patient is otherwise blind in both eyes.

Prognosis

- Guarded; depends on aggressiveness of the disease. Some patients respond well to treatment while others become progressively blind despite maximal therapy.

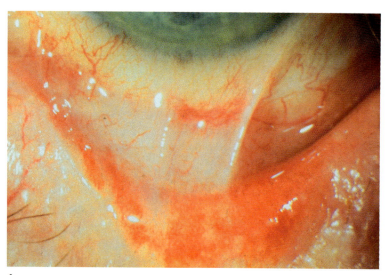

A

Figure 8-6 Ocular cicatricial pemphigoid A. *Forniceal foreshortening and early symblepharon formation can be seen in this patient with mild ocular cicatricial pemphigoid. The diagnosis was confirmed with a conjunctival biopsy and immunofluorescent stains. (Continued.)*

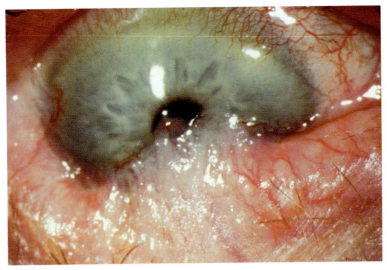

B

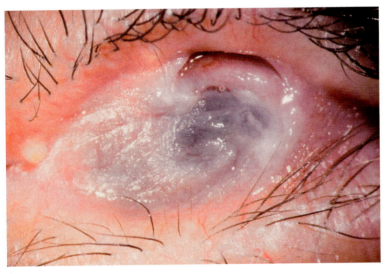

C

Figure 8-6 (cont.) Ocular cicatricial pemphigoid *B. Obliteration of the inferior fornix with severe, progressive scarring of the eyelid to the cornea is present in this patient with progressive ocular cicatricial pemphigoid. C. Total corneal scarring and keratinization occurred in this eye despite aggressive systemic treatment for ocular cicatricial pemphigoid. When both eyes are similarly involved, a permanent keratoprosthesis may be an option.*

STEVENS-JOHNSON SYNDROME (ERYTHEMA MULTIFORME MAJOR)

Stevens-Johnson syndrome is an acute, self-limited, inflammatory vesiculobullous disease of the skin and mucous membranes that is most frequently triggered by drugs or infections.

Etiology and Epidemiology

- It is caused by a type III hypersensitivity reaction in the dermis and conjunctival stroma that is potentially fatal (mortality rate, 10% to 33%) due to multisystem involvement.
- May affect all age groups but more common in young adults, and more common in females.

Causes
- Drugs: sulfonamides, penicillins, barbiturates, salicylates, anticonvulsants, others.
- Infections: herpes, mycoplasma, Coxsackie virus, echovirus, streptococcus, others.

Symptoms

- Acute onset of skin rash, ocular redness, discharge, foreign-body sensation, decreased vision
- May have a prodrome of headache, fever, malaise, arthralgias

Signs

- Bilateral diffuse conjunctivitis which may be associated with pseudomembranes
- Oral mucous membrane bullous erosions, hemorrhagic crusting of lips
- Skin lesions: diffuse erythema, classic "target" lesions, macular epidermal lesions, sloughing of skin (Figure 8-7A)
- Long-term sequelae include conjunctival fibrosis, symblepharon, distichiasis, trichiasis, punctal occlusion, dry eye, entropion, corneal neovascularization, keratinization of conjunctiva and cornea, persistent epithelial defect, melting, and perforation (Figures 8-7B,C)

Differential Diagnosis

- Ocular cicatricial pemphigoid: see above
- Toxic epidermal necrolysis: in young children, rare in adults
- Staphylococcal scalded skin syndrome: in young children, mucous membranes uninvolved.

Treatment

- Hospitalize the patient; may require treatment in a burn unit.
- Treat underlying infection or discontinue the offending medication.
- Topical corticosteroids (e.g., prednisolone 1% or dexamethasone 0.1%) drops q 2 to 6 h for 3 to 7 days. Need to monitor for epithelial defect and corneal thinning.
- Topical antibiotic ointment (e.g., erythromycin, bacitracin, or tetracycline) q 2 to 6 h.
- Artificial tear drops or ointments q 2 to 6 h.
- Break symblepharon daily with glass rod under topical anesthesia.
- Systemic corticosteroids are controversial.
- The long-term management of ocular complications is similar to that for ocular cicatricial pemphigoid.

Prognosis

- Good for mild cases, which may resolve with minimal sequelae. Moderate to severe cases can result in significant corneal and conjunctival damage with permanently decreased vision. Corneal transplants have a poor success rate.

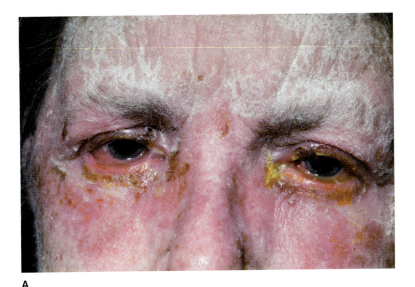

A

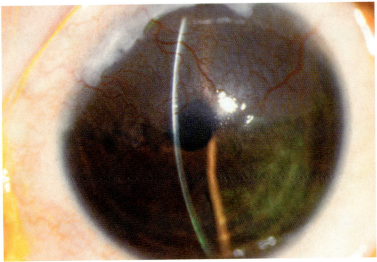

B

Figure 8-7   Stevens-Johnson syndrome   A. *This patient has severe scaling of the skin and a mucopurulent conjunctivitis due to Stevens-Johnson syndrome from phenytoin (Dilantin®).* **B.** *Significant superficial corneal scarring and neovascularization can be seen in this eye after an episode of Stevens-Johnson syndrome. (Continued.)*

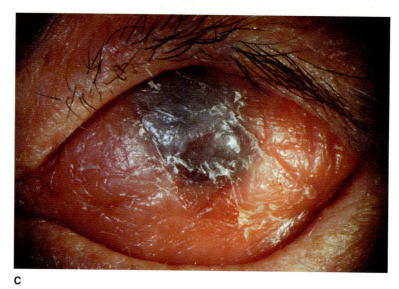

C

Figure 8-7 (cont.) Stevens-Johnson syndrome C. *End-stage corneal scarring and complete keratinization of the ocular surface is present in this eye after a severe case of Stevens-Johnson syndrome. When both eyes are similarly involved, a permanent keratoprosthesis may be an option.*

MOOREN'S ULCER

Mooren's ulcer is a rare, unilateral or bilateral, painful, inflammatory, chronic progressive ulcerative disease of the peripheral cornea. Two forms have been described. The first is a more benign unilateral condition in the elderly and the second is a bilateral affliction with relentless progression seen in younger males.

Etiology

- Idiopathic, by definition, but presumably immunologically based.
- A rare form related to hepatitis C infection has been identified.

Symptoms

- Redness, pain, photophobia, decreased vision, discharge

Signs

- Peripheral ulcerative keratitis with an epithelial defect. Typically begins nasally or temporally (Figure 8-8A).
- Ulcer extends circumferentially and centrally, with a leading undermined edge. The entire corneal circumference and the sclera may be involved in severe cases (Figure 8-8B).
- Perforation is uncommon but may occur in the progressive form.
- Healing takes place from the periphery, resulting in a thinned, vascularized cornea.

Differential Diagnosis

- Peripheral ulcerative keratitis associated with collagen vascular diseases: peripheral, unilateral or bilateral stromal infiltrates with thinning
- Staphylococcal hypersensitivity keratitis: multiple, usually bilateral stromal infiltrates with intact epithelium in early stages, and frequently associated with blepharitis and meibomitis
- Terrien's marginal degeneration: bilateral, painless, eye is not inflamed, epithelium is intact, thinning usually begins superiorly

Diagnosis

- This is made clinically, after excluding other causes of peripheral ulcerative keratitis.

Treatment

- Antibiotic ointment (e.g., polymyxin B/bacitracin, ciprofloxacin) q 2 to 6 h.
- Cycloplegics (e.g., scopolamine 0.5% or atropine 1% tid).
- Systemic corticosteroids (e.g., prednisolone 1 to 2 mg/kg po qd).
- Topical corticosteroids (e.g., prednisolone 1% or dexamethasone 0.1%) q 2 to 6 h. Frequency should be reduced or use should be discontinued if significant corneal thinning is encountered.
- Topical cyclosporine 1% to 2% q 2 to 6 h may have corticosteroid-sparing action.
- Topical collagenase inhibitors (e.g., acetylcysteine 10% drops qid) may be helpful.
- Systemic immunosuppressive agents (e.g., cyclosporine, methotrexate, cyclophosphamide) may be required with more severe disease.
- Conjunctival recession or resection with or without cryotherapy may reduce the stimuli for peripheral corneal inflammation.
- Lateral tarsorrhaphy, conjunctival autograft or amniotic membrane graft may be helpful in nonhealing epithelial defect and ulceration.
- Small perforations can be treated with cyanoacrylate tissue adhesive.
- Larger perforations or impending perforations may require lamellar or penetrating keratoplasty.
- When hepatitis C–related, consider treatment with alpha-interferon.

Prognosis

- Fair to good in the unilateral form, poor in the bilateral form.

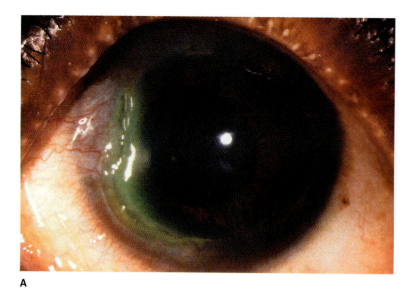

A

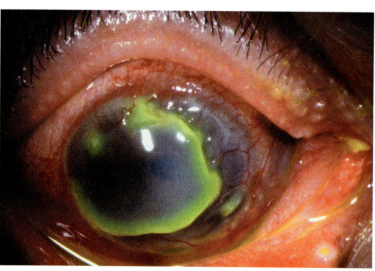

B

Figure 8-8   Mooren's ulcer   A. *Peripheral corneal ulceration from 6 to 10 o'clock, and also at 12 o'clock can be seen. Corneal scarring and neovascularization are present for almost 360 degrees from previous bouts of inflammation. This patient had bilateral Mooren's ulcers.* **B.** *This Mooren's ulcer has extended circumferentially for about 270 degrees. The peripheral cornea has healed with scarring and neovascularization, but an epithelial defect can be seen at the leading aspect of the ulceration, with an undermined ledge.*

PHLYCTENULOSIS

Phlyctenulosis is an uncommon, usually unilateral condition affecting the conjunctiva and/or cornea as a result of hypersensitivity type IV reaction to microbial antigens.

Etiology

- Staphylococcal infection: associated with blepharitis. Most common
- Tuberculosis
- Less common: *Chlamydia, Candida,* coccidioidomycosis

Symptoms

- Redness, foreign body sensation, pain, tearing, photophobia
- More severe when the cornea is involved, and may affect vision
- May have a history of multiple chalazia

Signs

- Small, round, elevated pinkish-white nodule which may involve the conjunctiva, limbus, or cornea. Usually based at the limbus (Figure 8-9).
- The phlycten may or may not have an epithelial defect.

Differential Diagnosis

- Inflamed pinguecula
- Rosacea keratitis
- Limbal herpes keratitis
- Microbial keratitis

Diagnosis

- Exclude underlying infection, especially tuberculosis.

Treatment

- Treat underlying infection and/or blepharitis if present.
- Antibiotic ointments (e.g., erythromycin or tetracycline) bid.
- Topical corticosteroids (e.g., prednisolone 1%, loteprednol 0.5%, or dexamethasone 0.1%) q 4 to 6 h.
- Cycloplegics (e.g., cyclopentolate 1% or scopolamine 0.25% tid).
- Oral tetracycline 250 mg po qid or doxycycline 100 mg po bid in severe cases associated with blepharitis. Children can be treated with erythromycin, approximately 200 mg po qd.
- Superficial keratectomy may occasionally be performed for corneal scars after resolution of the condition.

Prognosis

- Very good. May have residual corneal scarring and decreased vision.

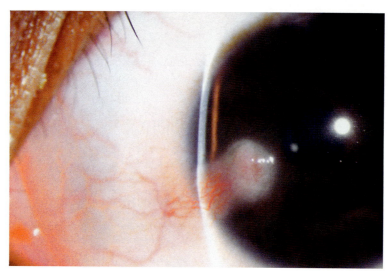

Figure 8-9 Phlyctenulosis *This elevated nodule with a neovascular leash from the limbus is classic for a corneal phlyctenule. It is typically due to eyelid disease such as blepharitis and staphylococcal hypersensitivity, but may be due to more serious infections such as tuberculosis.*

STAPHYLOCOCCAL HYPERSENSITIVITY

Staphylococcal hypersensitivity is a very common, transient, often bilateral condition that is associated with chronic staphylococcal blepharitis.

Etiology

- Hypersensitivity reaction to staphylococcal exotoxins or antigens

Symptoms

- Irritation, mild pain, redness, mild tearing, minimal to no discharge, history of previous episodes

Signs

- Begins as single or multiple, unilateral or bilateral, nonstaining, peripheral corneal infiltrates (Figure 8-10).
- These subepithelial/anterior stromal infiltrates are separated from the limbus by clear cornea.
- Infiltrates are usually found at the 2, 4, 8, and 10 o'clock positions of the peripheral cornea, where the eyelid margin crosses the limbus.
- Secondary epithelial breakdown is common.
- Resolves over a few days, leaving behind mild thinning, superficial vascularization, and peripheral scarring.

Differential Diagnosis

- See Mooren's Ulcer.
- In addition, consider infectious keratitis if symptoms are severe, infiltrate is located more centrally, an epithelial defect is present prior to or simultaneous with the onset of infiltrate, and if there is significant anterior chamber reaction.

Treatment

- Treat underlying blepharitis.
- Topical antibiotic ointment (e.g., erythromycin or tetracycline) bid.
- Topical corticosteroids (e.g., prednisolone 0.125% to 1%, loteprednol 0.2% to 0.5%, or fluorometholone 0.1%) qid once infection has been ruled out.

Prognosis

- Very good. Chronic treatment of blepharitis is typically required to prevent recurrences.

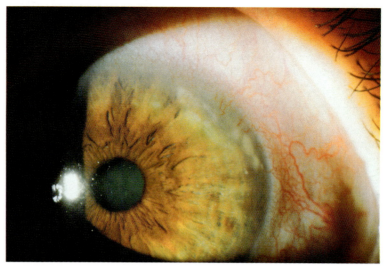

Figure 8-10 Staphylococcal hypersensitivity *Multiple creamy-white corneal infiltrates can be seen in the periphery from the 1 to 3 o'clock positions. There is a clear zone between the infiltrates and the limbus. Staphylococcal hypersensitivity infiltrates are most commonly located at the 2, 4, 8 and 10 o'clock positions, where the eyelid margin crosses the limbus.*

CORNEAL GRAFT REJECTION

Corneal allograft rejection is one of the leading causes of late graft failure after corneal transplantation.

Etiology

- Type IV hypersensitivity to major histocompatibility complex antigens present in donor cornea.

Symptoms

- Blurred vision, mild discomfort, redness, photophobia, irritation, but may be asymptomatic.
- Later, may have markedly decreased vision, irritation, pain, tearing.

Signs

- Circumcorneal conjunctival injection, anterior chamber reaction
- Subepithelial infiltrates (Krachmer's spots), epithelial rejection line, keratic precipitates, endothelial rejection line (Khodadoust's line) present in the donor cornea (Figures 8-11A,B,C,D)
- Epithelial or stromal edema, superficial or stromal neovascularization into the donor cornea (Figure 8-11E)

Differential Diagnosis

- Primary graft failure: graft edema present from the first postoperative day. Absence of white cell infiltration. This is usually due to poor quality of the donor cornea or intraoperative damage to the donor cornea.
- Reactivation of herpes keratitis: epithelial dendrite, stromal infiltrates, and keratic precipitates are present in both recipient and donor cornea. May worsen with topical corticosteroid therapy alone.
- Uveitis: may be confused with early graft rejection. When in doubt, treat as if rejection.
- Epithelial downgrowth: appears as advancing line with smooth or scalloped edges on both recipient and donor corneal endothelium, with minimal to no corneal edema. May grow onto the surface of iris. Progresses despite intense corticosteroid therapy.

Treatment

- Urgent therapy with topical corticosteroids (e.g., prednisolone 1% or dexamethasone 0.1%) q 1 h for a week during waking hours and taper to qid by 3 to 4 weeks. Corticosteroid ointment qhs may be used in addition.
- Topical cyclosporine 1% to 2% q 2 to 6 h can be added.
- Systemic corticosteroids (e.g., prednisolone 1 mg/kg/d po qd) for 2 weeks and then tapered over 1 week may be considered if there is a lack of response to topical therapy or for recurrent rejection. Alternatively, patient can be hospitalized for a single-dose methylprednisolone 500 mg IV infusion given over a few hours.
- Topical cycloplegics (e.g., cyclopentolate 1% or scopolamine 0.25% bid) if significant iritis is present.
- Topical antibiotic prophylaxis (e.g., erythromycin, bacitracin, or tetracycline ointment bid to qhs).

Prognosis

- Very good if diagnosed and treated within a few days, poor if treatment is delayed more than 1 to 2 weeks.

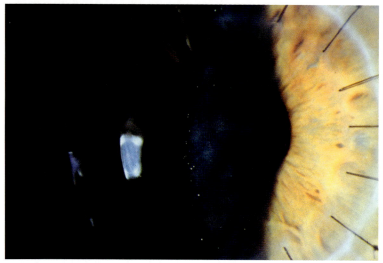

A

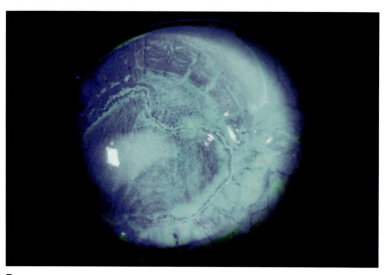

B

Figure 8-11 Corneal graft rejection **A.** *Multiple subepithelial infiltrates are present in this corneal transplant. Originally thought to represent postviral infiltrates, they are really evidence of mild graft rejection. While they typically do not cause significant damage to the graft or decrease vision, they are often harbingers of more severe forms or rejection, such as endothelial rejection, which can significantly harm the transplant.* **B.** *A raised curvilinear epithelial line, which stains faintly, can be seen near the periphery of the corneal graft winding around from the 10 to 6 o'clock positions. This represents an epithelial rejection line, the battle line between the donor and host epithelium. This type of rejection is also typically not graft- or vision-threatening, but indicates an active immune response with an increased risk of more severe rejection. (Continued.)*

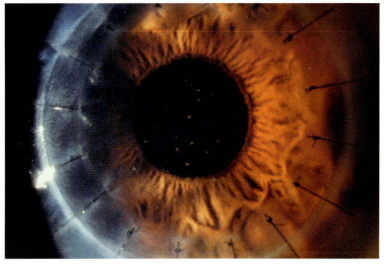

C

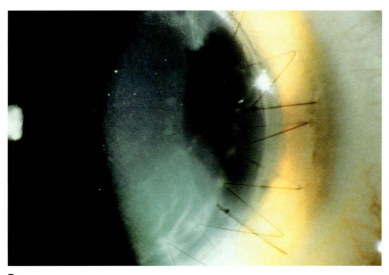

D

Figure 8-11 (cont.) **Corneal graft rejection** C. *Numerous pigmented keratic precipitates are visible on the endothelial surface of this corneal graft. Slight corneal haze indicating mild corneal edema is also seen. New keratic precipitates represent endothelial rejection. The corneal edema indicates some endothelial compromise. Endothelial rejection needs to be treated aggressively to preserve as much healthy endothelium as possible.* **D.** *A line of keratic precipitates can be seen extending from the 2 to 7 o'clock positions, which is an endothelial rejection line (Khodadoust's line). Such lines tend to move from the corneal periphery toward the center of the cornea and can cross the entire cornea. Note the corneal edema peripheral to this endothelial rejection line. Endothelial rejection lines require aggressive antirejection treatment. (Continued.)*

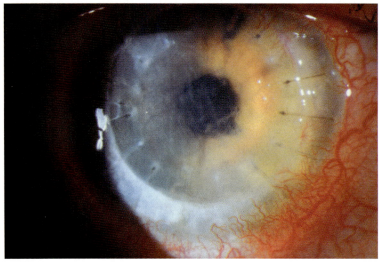

E

Figure 8-11 (cont.) **Corneal graft rejection** **E.** *Severe diffuse corneal edema with multiple keratic precipitates (some in a linear pattern at the inferior edge of the pupil) indicates advanced endothelial rejection. There is often associated conjunctival injection and iritis. Treatment is with intensive topical and occasionally systemic corticosteroids to spare as many endothelial cells as possible.*

Chapter 9

ANTERIOR SCLERA AND IRIS

EPISCLERITIS

Episcleritis is a benign, transient, recurrent, self-limited and usually nonspecific condition affecting young adults. It rarely progresses to scleritis, and should not be considered as a milder form of scleritis.

Etiology

- Idiopathic
- Collagen vascular diseases
- Rosacea
- Gout
- Herpes zoster, herpes simplex, syphilis

Symptoms

- Acute onset of redness, mild irritation, tearing

Signs

There are two forms: simple and nodular episcleritis.

Simple Episcleritis
- Sectorial or diffuse hyperemia, primarily involving the middle episcleral plexus, with some secondary involvement of the overlying conjunctival vessels (Figures 9-1A,B).
- The inflamed episcleral vessels have a straight, radial configuration.
- Topical phenylephrine 2.5% will cause blanching and enhance visualization of the normal deep vascular plexus over the sclera.

Nodular Episcleritis
- Somewhat tender, usually solitary, localized injected nodule which can be moved slightly over the sclera.

- A localized area of corneal thinning secondary to desiccation (delle) may develop adjacent to the episcleral nodule.

Differential Diagnosis

- Conjunctivitis: usually associated with papillary or follicular response in the tarsal conjunctiva. May have a mucoid or purulent discharge.
- Scleritis: pain is deeper and more severe, sclera has a purple or bluish hue under natural light, injected scleral vessels have criss-crossing configuration, vessels are immobile over the globe, patients tend to be older.
- Inflamed pinguecula: located in the completely mobile conjunctiva.

Diagnosis

- Examination is made with the slit-lamp and under natural or room lights.
- Attempt to move the episcleral vessels over the sclera using a cotton-tipped stick under topical anesthesia.
- Apply phenylephrine 2.5% and observe for blanching of episcleral vessels after 15 minutes.
- Systemic work-up if history is suggestive of collagen vascular disease or gout.

Treatment

- Artificial tears and cool compresses qid.
- Consider a short course of topical antihistamine drops (e.g., tetrahydrozoline, naphazoline, or antazoline tid).
- Consider a short course of a topical non-steroidal anti-inflammatory agent (NSAID) (e.g., diclofenac, ketorolac, or ibuprofen qid).
- Oral NSAID (e.g., indomethacin 12.5 to 25 mg qd to tid or flurbiprofen 100 mg bid to tid) for moderate to severe cases.
- Consider a short course of topical corticosteroids (e.g., fluorometholone 0.1 to 0.25%, loteprednol 0.2 to 0.5%) qid in recalcitrant cases.

Prognosis

- Good to very good. Episcleritis is often a recurrent condition.

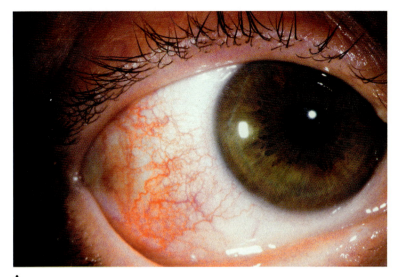

A

B

Figure 9-1 Episcleritis **A.** *Localized injection of the episcleral vessels is evident in this patient with sectorial episcleritis.* **B.** *Diffuse injection of the episcleral vessels is present in this eye. Episcleritis can be difficult to differentiate from scleritis in certain patients. Episcleral vessels tend to blanch with topical phenylephrine 2.5% while scleral vessels do not.*

ANTERIOR SCLERITIS

Scleritis is a severe, potentially sight-threatening ocular disorder that carries a totally different prognosis than episcleritis. It may be mild and benign or severe and destructive. Females are affected more often than males and the condition is frequently bilateral. The majority of scleritis affects the anterior sclera. Scleritis can be further divided into the following clinical forms:

NONNECROTIZING SCLERITIS

- **Diffuse** Diffuse hyperemia and distortion of the pattern of the deep vascular plexus, associated with variable episcleral and conjunctival injection (Figure 9-2A). This is the most benign form associated with the least severe systemic conditions.

- **Nodular** Tender, usually solitary, deep, localized injected nodule which cannot be moved over the sclera (Figure 9-2B).

NECROTIZING SCLERITIS

- **With Inflammation**
  — This is the most destructive form of scleritis. It is associated with ocular or systemic complications in 60% of patients and 40% may have loss of vision. One third of patients may die within a few years as a result of severe autoimmune disease if inadequately treated.
  — Gradual appearance of painful, localized, avascular patch overlying an area of scleral necrosis (Figure 9-2C).
  — Inflammation may be localized to the surrounding sclera or become diffuse.
  — The underlying uvea progressively becomes visible through the thinned and necrotic sclera.

- **Without Inflammation (Scleromalacia Perforans)**
  — Typically seen in patients with long-standing rheumatoid arthritis.
  — Asymptomatic development of enlarging gray-blue patches of scleral thinning.
  — Exposure of underlying uvea through areas of thin, devitalized sclera with large bridging vessels.
  — Anterior scleral staphylomas can occur.

Etiology

- Half of the patients with scleritis have an associated systemic disease.

Idiopathic

Iatrogenic
- Surgery (e.g., cataract surgery, trabeculectomy, scleral buckle) (Figure 9-2D)
- Topical medications (e.g., NSAIDs, corticosteroids) (Figure 9-2E)

Collagen Vascular Diseases
- Rheumatoid arthritis (most common)
- Wegener's granulomatosis (moderately common)
- Polyarteritis nodosa
- Relapsing polychondritis
- Others (e.g., systemic lupus erythematosus, juvenile rheumatoid arthritis, juvenile chronic arthritis, polymyositis)

Granulomatous Diseases
- Sarcoidosis
- Tuberculosis
- Syphilis
- Lyme disease

Skin Diseases
- Herpes zoster ophthalmicus (moderately common)
- Acne rosacea

Gout

Complications of Scleritis

- Stromal keratitis, peripheral corneal melt and sclerosing keratitis, associated with worse prognosis
- Uveitis
- Cataract
- Glaucoma
- Posterior uveitis, posterior scleritis, exudative retinal detachment

Symptoms

- Severe, boring pain that may radiate to the orbit or head and awaken patients from sleep, redness, tearing, photophobia, decreased vision.
- Onset is generally gradual, but may be acute.
- History of associated systemic diseases in many cases.

Signs

- Inflamed conjunctiva, episclera, and sclera. Scleral vessels have criss-crossing patterns, do not blanch with 2.5% phenylephrine drops, and are immobile over the globe.
- Sclera has a purple-bluish hue when examined grossly under natural light.
- Scleral inflammation can be sectorial or diffuse. Scleral edema, nodule, or thinning and necrosis may be seen. Sometimes, the sclera may become more translucent without significant thinning.
- Anterior chamber reaction.
- Other signs of ocular complications as mentioned above may be observed.

Differential Diagnosis

- Episcleritis
- Inflamed pinguecula
- Infectious scleritis

Diagnosis

- Examination at the slit-lamp and under natural or room lights.

- Attempt to move the injected vessels over the sclera using a cotton-tipped stick under topical anesthesia.
- Apply phenylephrine 2.5% and observe for absence of blanching of the scleral vessels after 15 minutes.
- Investigate for associated systemic diseases.

Treatment

For nonnecrotizing diffuse and nodular scleritis:

- Oral NSAIDs (e.g., indomethacin 25 mg tid or flurbiprofen 100 mg tid) are often effective.
- For more resistant cases, systemic corticosteroids (e.g., prednisolone 1 to 2 mg/kg/d po qd), then tapered over the next few months.

For necrotizing scleritis:

- Oral NSAIDs for 1 week.
- If there is no improvement, systemic corticosteroid is added as above.
- For very severe disease, the patient can be hospitalized and given IV corticosteroids.
- In resistant cases, other immunosuppressive therapy may be indicated (e.g., methotrexate, cyclophosphamide, azathioprine, and cyclosporine).
- Scleral (or pericardial or dural) patch graft may be required if there is a risk of perforation.
- Topical corticosteroids are not effective for scleritis. Topical cyclosporine 2% drops, 4 to 6 per day, may be of limited benefit.
- Subtenon's corticosteroid injections are typically contraindicated as they may cause scleral thinning and may increase the risk of perforation.

Prognosis

- Good for nonnecrotizing scleritis, guarded for necrotizing scleritis. The prognosis depends greatly on whether the underlying systemic disease can be identified and treated adequately.

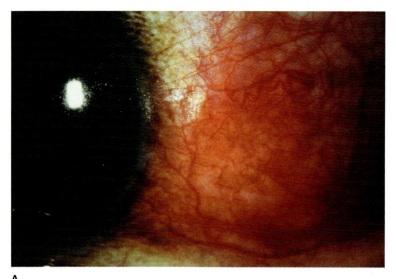

A

B

Figure 9-2   Scleritis   A. *Diffuse inflammation of the conjunctiva and sclera is present in this eye with diffuse scleritis. The vessels did not blanch with topical phenylephrine 2.5%.* **B.** *An elevated, inflamed nodule of sclera can be seen. A purplish hue is present deep to the prominent vessels, suggesting scleral inflammation. (Continued.)*

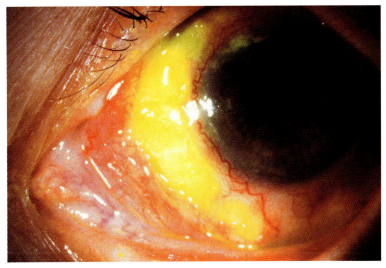

C

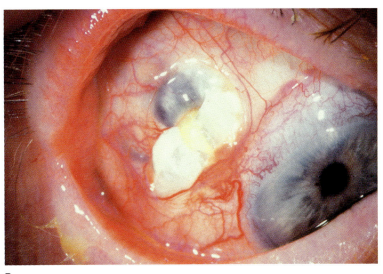

D

Figure 9-2 (cont.) **Necrotizing scleritis** **C.** *A large area of necrotizing scleritis with peripheral corneal involvement can be seen in this patient with presumed Wegener's granulomatosis. Multiple scleral patch grafts, amniotic membrane grafts, and treatment with numerous systemic immunosuppressive agents failed to reverse the progression of this condition which eventually resulted in enucleation.* **D.** *An exposed scleral buckle has resulted in scleral melting with uveal show. It was treated with removal of the encircling band and a scleral patch graft. (Continued.)*

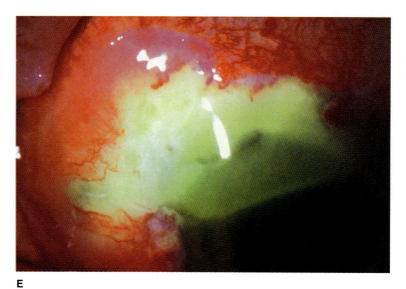

E

Figure 9-2 (cont.)   Corneoscleral melt   E. *Ten days after limbal cataract surgery treated postoperatively with topical corticosteroids and generic diclofenac, a severe corneoscleral melt developed. Cultures were negative and the condition did not improve with intensive topical fortified antibiotics. Two days later it perforated requiring a large corneoscleral graft (see Figure 10-10B).*

IRIS CYSTS

IRIS PIGMENT EPITHELIAL CYST

- More common than iris stromal cysts.
- Arise from the posterior pigment epithelial layer of the iris.
- Note a smooth, dome-shaped iris elevation (Figure 9-3A).
- Often distinguishable from a solid iris lesion with transillumination or ultrasound biomicroscopy.
- Rarely, iris pigment epithelial cysts can detach and become free-floating, at which point they can be removed. Otherwise, they are followed.

IRIS STROMAL CYST

- Less common than iris pigment epithelial cysts.
- Arise from the iris stroma.
- Note a thin, translucent cyst wall that can occupy a large portion of the anterior chamber (Figure 9-3B).
- Generally followed unless obscuring vision, in which case they can be treated with aspiration, cryotherapy, or laser treatment or excision, but they can recur or develop sheetlike epithelial downgrowth.

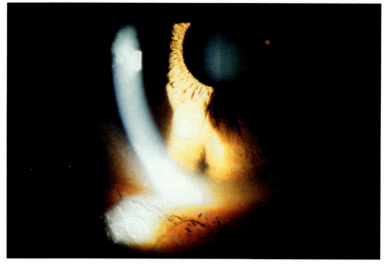

A

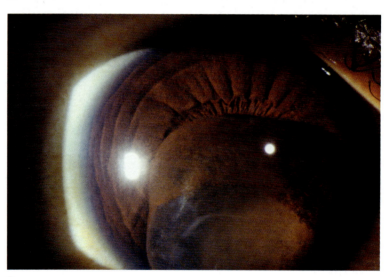

B

Figure 9-3   Iris pigment epithelial cyst   A. *An elevation in the peripheral iris can be seen at the 6:30 position. Ultrasound biomicroscopy revealed an iris pigment epithelial cyst pushing the iris stroma forward. It often looks like a "rug draped over a ball."* **Iris stromal cyst   B.** *This large thin-walled cyst of the iris stroma was so large it covered the pupil. Remarkably, the vision was approximately 20/60 at this time. There was no history of ocular trauma or surgery.*

IRIS TUMORS

IRIS NEVUS

- Flat or minimally elevated hyperpigmented lesion on the iris surface (Figure 9-4A).
- Often appear or enlarge slightly during puberty.
- Generally do not grow.
- Management is with documentation of size and observation.

MALIGNANT MELANOMA

- May be localized or diffuse
- May be pigmented or nonpigmented
- Most important sign is documented growth
- May require excisional biopsy, more extensive surgery radiation therapy, or enucleation

METASTATIC TUMOR

- Tend to be amelanotic (Figure 9-4B).
- Tend to have multiple lesions in both eyes.
- May have tumor cells in the anterior chamber with a pseudohypopyon.
- Most commonly from lung cancer in males and breast cancer in women.
- Systemic treatment for the primary cancer is indicated.
- Iris tumors may respond to local radiation and systemic chemotherapy.

VASCULAR TUMOR

- Rare (Figure 9-4C).

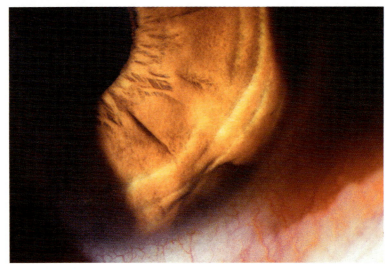

A

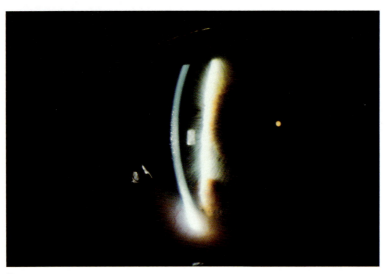

B

Figure 9-4 Iris nevus A. *This smooth, round pigmented iris mass, which did not involve the anterior chamber angle, is an iris nevus. Iris nevi need to be followed routinely for evidence of growth.* **Iris tumor B.** *A pigmented mass on the iris surface is evident in this patient with metastatic lung cancer. It was thought to be a metastatic tumor to the iris. (Continued.)*

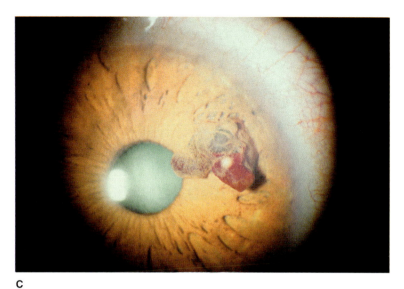

C

Figure 9-4 (cont.)   Iris vascular tumor   *C. A large multilobed vascular iris lesion is present. It was resected due to intermittent bleeding.*

Chapter 10

SURGERY AND COMPLICATIONS

CATARACT EXTRACTION AND INTRAOCULAR LENS IMPLANTATION

Cataract extraction and intraocular lens (IOL) implantation involves removal of a cloudy crystalline lens and replacement with an artificial lens. It is one of the most commonly performed surgical procedures.

Indications

- Visually significant lens opacity
- Rarely, a cataract causing intraocular inflammation and/or glaucoma

Surgical Technique

Anesthesia Topical or local.

Extracapsular Method A large limbal incision is made near the limbus, an anterior capsulotomy is performed, the lens nucleus is prolapsed out of the eye, the residual cortical material is removed, an IOL is placed, and the wound is sutured.

Phacoemulsification Method A small limbal or clear corneal incision is made, an anterior capsulotomy is performed, the lens nucleus is fragmented and removed with an ultrasound probe, the residual cortical material is removed, and an IOL is placed. Often, no sutures are required.

Postoperative Management Topical corticosteroid and antibiotics.

Complications

Intraoperative
- Expulsive hemorrhage
- Vitreous prolapse
- Lens material falls into posterior segment
- Phacoemulsification burn (Figure 10-1A)

Postoperative
- Endophthalmitis
- Wound leak, wound infection
- Cystoid macular edema
- Glaucoma
- Retinal detachment
- IOL subluxation or dislocation; pupillary capture of IOL (Figures 10-1B,C,D)
- Traumatic wound rupture
- Posterior capsular opacity (PCO), very common (Figure 10-1E)

Success Rate

- Excellent. PCO may require a laser capsulotomy.

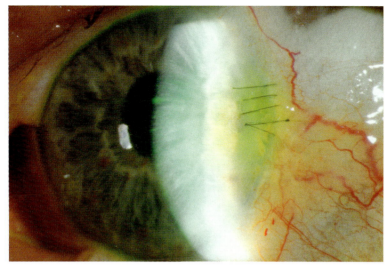

A

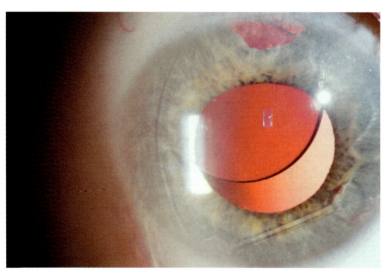

B

Figure 10-1 Phacoemulsification burn A. *This eye withstood a phacoemulsification burn during temporal clear corneal cataract surgery. A phacoemulsification burn during cataract surgery is caused, at least in part, by inadequate cooling of the phacoemulsification handpiece tip during use, causing a thermal burn at the wound. It can occur very quickly, within seconds. The wound required 5 sutures to close. There are significant corneal striae due to the tightness of the sutures required to keep the wound watertight.* **Intraocular lens subluxation B.** *This anterior chamber intraocular lens is superiorly subluxed. The superior haptic has migrated through the superior peripheral iridectomy allowing the inferior haptic to come out of the angle and intermittently contact the inferior corneal endothelium, causing corneal edema. (Continued.)*

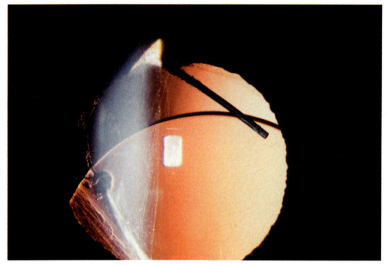

C

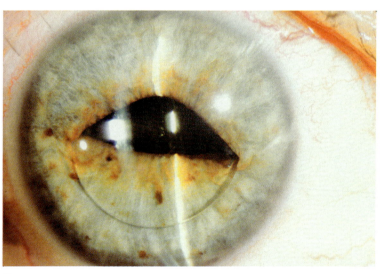

D

Figure 10-1 (cont.)   Intraocular lens subluxation   C. *This posterior chamber intraocular lens has subluxed inferiorly. An oblique rent in the posterior capsule can be seen, compromising capsular support. An inferior subluxation is often termed a "sunset syndrome."* **Pupillary capture D.** *This posterior chamber intraocular lens is partially captured by the iris in this eye 2 weeks after cataract surgery. It was repositioned in the posterior chamber in the operating room. (Continued.)*

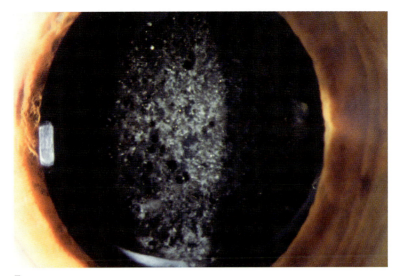

E

Figure 10-1 (cont.)   Posterior capsular opacity   E. *A moderate posterior capsular opacity is evident in this eye several years after cataract surgery. Fibrosis of the initially clear posterior capsule often occurs after cataract surgery and can affect visual clarity. Note the arc of opacified anterior capsular rim inferiorly and the fibrotic posterior capsule centrally. When this affects visual function, treatment is with a laser capsulotomy.*

CORNEAL TRANSPLANTATION (PENETRATING KERATOPLASTY)

Penetrating keratoplasty involves removal of diseased host tissue and replacing it with full-thickness normal donor cornea. It is one of the most successful transplant operations today, depending on the primary corneal disease.

Indications

Optical   To improve vision.

Tectonic   To restore the structural integrity of the eye.

Therapeutic   Usually performed to remove infected and/or perforated corneal tissue that is not responsive to medical treatment.

Pain   To improve pain from chronic bullous keratopathy.

Cosmetic   To restore a more normal appearance to the eye.

- Most common indications for penetrating keratoplasty are aphakic or pseudophakic bullous keratopathy, regrafts, keratoconus, corneal dystrophies, and infectious and traumatic corneal scarring.

Donor Tissue

Contraindications for use as donor cornea:

- Death of unknown cause
- Death from central nervous system diseases of unknown etiology
- Central nervous system infections (e.g., Creutzfeldt-Jakob disease, subacute sclerosing panencephalitis, progressive multifocal leukoencephalopathy)
- Systemic infections (e.g., AIDS, viral hepatitis, rabies, septicemia, cytomegalovirus infection)
- Reye's syndrome
- Lymphoma and leukemia

Unfavorable Prognostic Factors

- Severe stromal vascularization
- Previous graft rejection

- Decreased corneal sensation (e.g., herpes keratitis)
- Pediatric patients
- Active uveitis
- Significant anterior synechiae
- Uncontrolled glaucoma
- Active corneal or intraocular infection
- Severe dry eyes
- Ocular surface inflammation, cicatrization, and keratinization
- Significant limbal stem cell deficiency
- Extreme thinning or irregularity at the intended graft-host junction
- Eyelid disorders: ectropion, entropion, exposure

Surgical Technique

Anesthesia   Local or general anesthesia.

Preparation of Operative Eye   Often, placement of a Flieringa ring helps to stabilize the globe.

Determination of Graft Size   Routine graft sizes vary from 7.25 mm to 8.5 mm.

Trephination of Donor Cornea   Typically performed using a posterior endothelial punch method. The trephine is usually 0.25 to 0.5 mm larger than that for host cornea trephination.

Excision of Host Cornea   Trephination of host cornea can be done by using a manual trephine (e.g., Weck trephine) or a vacuum trephine (e.g., Barron-Hessburg or Hanna trephine). A partial-thickness trephination is first carried out, the anterior chamber is then entered using a blade, and finally excision is completed using corneal scissors.

Wound Closure   Various suture methods, including interrupted, running, double running, or a combination may be used. 10-0 nylon is usually used (Figures 10-2A,B,C).

Postoperative Management   Topical corticosteroid and antibiotics.

Combined Procedures

Where indicated, penetrating keratoplasty can be combined with any of the following procedures:

- Cataract extraction with intraocular lens implantation (triple procedure)
- Anterior vitrectomy with intraocular lens implantation
- Intraocular lens exchange, either anterior chamber lens or scleral fixated posterior chamber lens
- Glaucoma drainage devices or trabeculectomy
- Posterior vitrectomy, possibly with a temporary keratoprosthesis

Complications

Intraoperative
- Eccentric, tilted, or irregular trephination of host or donor cornea
- Damage to iris or lens
- Expulsive hemorrhage
- Vitreous prolapse

Postoperative

SIGHT-THREATENING
- Endophthalmitis (Figure 10-2D)
- Glaucoma
- Retinal detachment
- Cataract
- Cystoid macular edema

GRAFT-THREATENING
- Primary failure: endothelial damage during surgery, poor quality donor tissue (Figure 10-2E)
- Wound leak (Figure 10-2F)
- Persistent epithelial defect (Figure 10-2G)
- Flat anterior chamber (typically from a wound leak or angle-closure glaucoma)
- Immunologic rejection
- Infectious keratitis, suture abscess (Figure 10-2H)
- Recurrence of disease: dystrophies, infection
- Epithelial downgrowth and retrocorneal fibrous membrane (Figure 10-2I)
- Vitreous touch

OTHERS
- Broken suture (Figures 10-2J,K)
- Iris prolapse
- Wound dehiscence
- Traumatic wound rupture (Figure 10-2l)
- Irregular astigmatism

Success Rate

- Poor to excellent, depending on the indication for surgery.

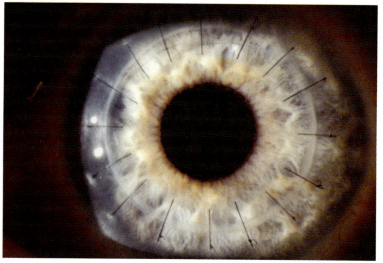

A

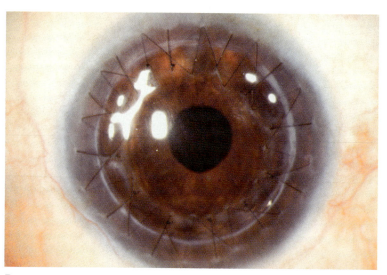

B

Figure 10-2 Corneal transplant *A. A clear corneal transplant is seen 6 weeks after surgery for herpes simplex scarring. Sixteen interrupted 10-0 nylon sutures are in place. B. A clear corneal transplant is seen 6 months after a corneal transplant, cataract extraction, and posterior chamber intraocular lens implant for Fuchs' dystrophy and cataract. Twelve interrupted and 12 bite running 10-0 nylon sutures are present. (Continued.)*

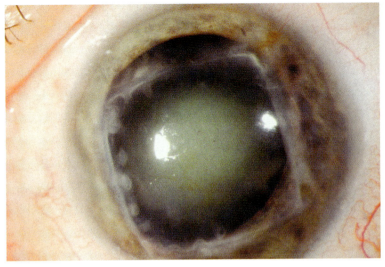

C

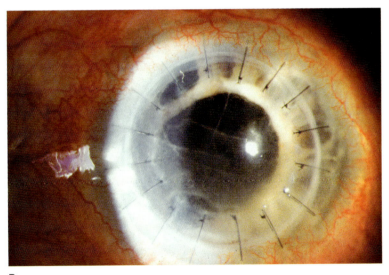

D

Figure 10-2 (cont.) Corneal transplant **C.** *An old square corneal transplant performed by Dr. Castroviejo in New York City about 40 years earlier. The graft remains remarkably clear, although a cataract is developing.* **Corneal transplant complication—early endophthalmitis D.** *Ten days after a corneal transplant, severe intraocular inflammation with fibrin in the anterior chamber and a small hypopyon at the graft-host margin inferiorly can be seen. Endophthalmitis was suspected and a vitreous tap revealed Staphylococcus epidermidis which responded well to antibiotic treatment. (Continued.)*

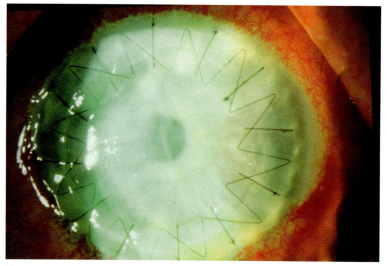

E

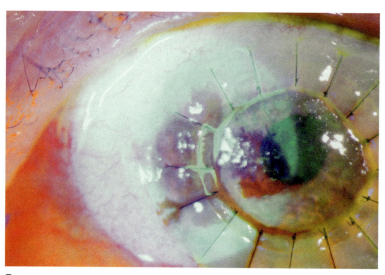

F

Figure 10-2 (cont.) Corneal transplant complication—primary graft failure **E.** *Diffuse severe corneal edema with whitening of the corneal stroma is present 1 day after a corneal transplant in an eye with primary graft failure. Primary graft failure generally occurs due to poor-quality tissue or damage to the corneal endothelium during surgery.* **Corneal transplant complication—wound leak** **F.** *A wound leak is seen 3 days after a corneal transplant. Dark, concentrated fluorescein dye was placed at the graft–host margin at the 9 o'clock position. Aqueous fluid leaking through the graft–host wound can be seen to dilute the dye and turn it bright yellow-green. If the leak is minimal and the anterior chamber is formed, it can be treated medically and followed closely. If the leak is significant or the chamber is flat, the leak should be repaired surgically. (Continued.)*

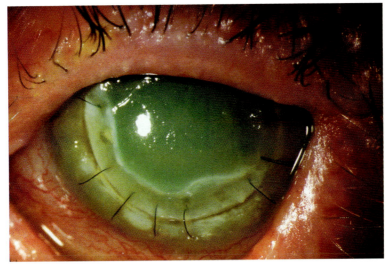

G

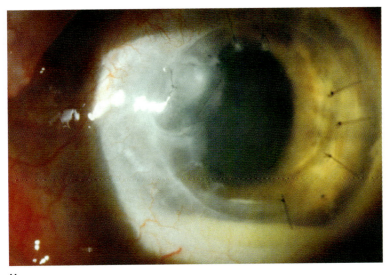

H

Figure 10-2 (cont.) **Corneal transplant complication—wound melt** **G.** *A severe corneal wound melt is present in the inferior half of this cornea 5 months after a corneal transplant. Multiple loose sutures can be seen. A small, permanent lateral tarsorrhaphy had already been performed.* **Corneal transplant complication—suture abscess** **H.** *A broken corneal transplant suture and underlying abscess are present at the 10 o'clock position. A large hypopyon with a second small hypopyon at the graft–host junction can be seen inferiorly. (Continued.)*

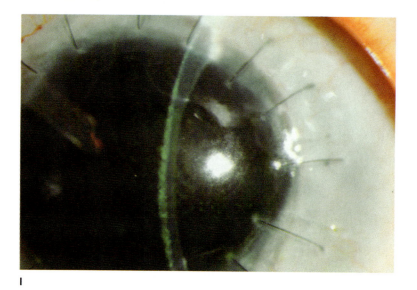

I

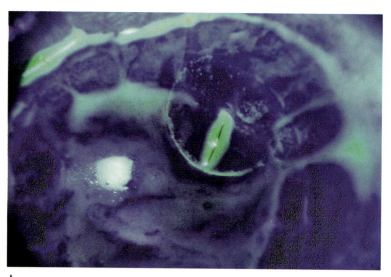

J

Figure 10-2 (cont.)   Corneal transplant complication—epithelial downgrowth   *I. A curvilinear retrocorneal membrane can be seen from 9 o'clock toward 12 o'clock and back down toward 3 o'clock. It is again visible around 5 o'clock. It advanced centrally over several weeks. It was diagnosed as epithelial downgrowth.* **Corneal transplant complication—broken interrupted suture**   *J. A broken corneal transplant suture is present at the 2 o'clock position. Fluorescein dye and the cobalt blue light demonstrate the "windshield wiper" effect of the broken suture. (Continued.)*

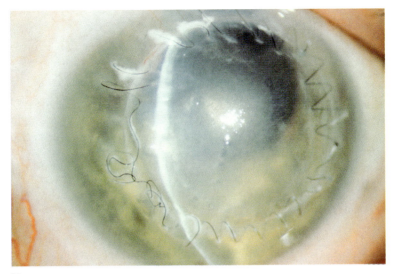

K

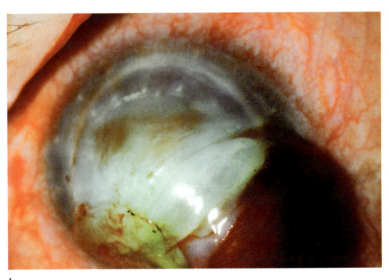

L

Figure 10-2 (cont.)   Corneal transplant complication—loose, exposed running suture
K. *An extremely loose and exposed running suture can be seen a year after a corneal transplant. There is mucus adherent to the suture and secondary peripheral corneal neovascularization superiorly and corneal edema centrally.* **Expulsive hemorrhage after a corneal transplant wound dehiscence   L.** *Several years after a penetrating keratoplasty, blunt trauma caused the wound to dehisce and resulted in an expulsive hemorrhage. Note the large clot of blood exiting the wound. Iris pigment and vitreous jelly can be seen on the inferior cornea.*

LAMELLAR KERATOPLASTY

Lamellar keratoplasty involves removal of the anterior cornea and replacing it with partial-thickness normal donor cornea.

Advantages

- Donor endothelial cell density is not important.
- The anterior chamber is not entered, therefore complications such as expulsive hemorrhage and endophthalmitis are avoided.
- No risk of endothelial rejection.

Disadvantages

- Technical complexity of the procedure.
- Opacification of the lamellar interface which may reduce visual acuity.

Indications

- Anterior corneal scars and dystrophies
- Recurrent pterygium
- Limbal dermoid
- Peripheral ulcerative keratitis
- Terrien's marginal degeneration
- Rarely, keratoconus, infectious keratitis, superficial corneal tumors

Surgical Technique

Anesthesia   Local or general anesthesia.
- Partial thickness corneal trephination (encompassing the pathology) is performed on the recipient cornea.
- Lamellar dissection is then carried out on the recipient cornea using a blunt dissecting blade.

- Donor lamellar cornea is dissected and trephined. It should be 0.25 to 0.5 mm larger than the recipient bed. Either a whole eye or a corneoscleral button fixated in an artificial chamber can be used.
- Alternatively, an automated microkeratome or a femtosecond laser can be used to dissect both the donor and recipient cornea.
- The recipient bed is irrigated to remove epithelium, debris, and blood, and the donor cornea is sutured with 10-0 nylon using either interrupted or running sutures (Figure 10-3).

Postoperative Management   Topical corticosteroid and antibiotics.

Complications

- Perforation of recipient or donor cornea during dissection, with possible need to convert to a penetrating keratoplasty
- Opacification of lamellar interface
- Irregular astigmatism
- Recurrence of disease: dystrophies, infection
- Persistent epithelial defect
- Fibrovascular ingrowth into lamellar interface
- Broken suture
- Infectious keratitis
- Stromal rejection (rare)

Success Rate

- Poor to very good, depending on the indication for surgery.

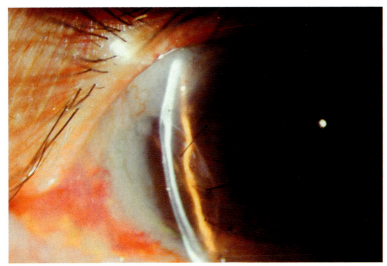

Figure 10-3 Lamellar keratoplasty *A lamellar keratoplasty was performed in this eye with a large recurrent pterygium associated with significant corneal scarring. The slit-lamp beam shows the deep lamellar incision. Multiple 10-0 nylon sutures are still in place.*

CORNEAL BIOPSY

The corneal biopsy procedure involves excision of a small disc of corneal tissue, usually of one- to two-thirds depth, for microbial or histologic examination.

Indications

- Presumed microbial keratitis that is culture negative and does not respond to medical therapy (e.g., *Acanthamoeba* or fungal keratitis)
- Ocular surface tumors (e.g., conjunctival intraepithelial neoplasia, squamous cell carcinoma), rarely

Surgical Technique

- Antimicrobials may be discontinued 24 hours prior to the procedure.
- Topical or local anesthesia can be used.
- Debris over the lesion is debrided and plated onto culture media in eyes with suspected infection.
- A site away from the visual axis and at the edge of the pathology is chosen, and a partial-thickness trephination to encompass the pathology using a 2-, 3-, or 4-mm diameter trephine is done. Lamellar dissection is completed with a blade (Figure 10-4).
- Infected tissue obtained is cut in half and sent for culture and histology.
- It may be wise to have donor tissue on standby for deep biopsy or for biopsy of necrotic lesions in case of perforation.

Complications

- Perforation
- Corneal scarring and irregularity

Success Rate

- Fair to good for determining the cause of the problem.

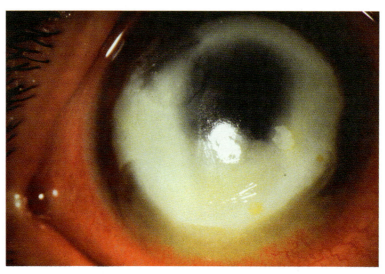

Figure 10-4 Corneal biopsy *A 3-mm diameter circular corneal biopsy site can be seen superotemporally in this right eye with a progressive corneal ulcer not responding to aggressive antibiotic medications. Half of the biopsy specimen was sent for histopathologic examination and the other half was sent for microbiologic evaluation.*

SUPERFICIAL KERATECTOMY

The superficial keratectomy procedure involves excision of the epithelium, Bowman's layer, and superficial stroma.

Indications

- Anterior corneal lesions (e.g., dermoid, ptery-gium, Salzmann's nodule, anterior basement membrane [ABM] dystrophy)
- For biopsy purposes
- Excision of tumors (e.g., squamous cell carci-noma), rarely

Surgical Technique

- Topical or local anesthesia may be used.
- The area of pathology is identified and marked.
- Superficial lamellar dissection is carried out using a blunt or sharp blade (Figure 10-5).
- After excision, the stromal bed can be smoothed with a diamond burr.

Complications

- Corneal haze or scar
- Residual opacity/pathology
- Irregular astigmatism

Prognosis

- Good to excellent, depending on the indica-tion and severity of the condition.

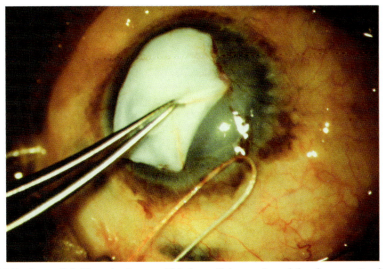

Figure 10-5 Superficial keratectomy *This large Salzmann's nodular degeneration lesion was removed with a blade, peeling it off of Bowman's membrane. The underlying cornea was remarkably clear. An advantage to peeling lesions off with a blade is that anatomic planes, such as Bowman's membrane, can be retained, potentially resulting in a smooth surface.*

EXCIMER LASER PHOTOTHERAPEUTIC KERATECTOMY (PTK)

Laser phototherapeutic keratectomy (PTK) involves using the excimer laser to ablate the anterior stroma with or without the overlying epithelium, to remove superficial irregularities and/or opacities.

Indications

- Anterior corneal dystrophies (e.g., ABM or Reis-Bücklers' dystrophies)
- Stromal dystrophies (e.g., superficial granular or lattice dystrophy)
- Superficial scars or nodules (e.g., Salzmann's nodular degeneration, keratoconus nodule, after pterygium surgery)
- Recurrent corneal erosions (traumatic or related to dystrophies)

Surgical Technique

- Topical anesthesia is used.
- Epithelium is removed using a blunt blade or by laser ablation.
- Laser ablation is carried out on the stroma with the patient maintaining steady fixation (Figures 10-6A,B).
- The ablation technique varies according to the pathology being treated.
- A masking agent (artificial tears) can be used during ablation to correct surface irregularities.

- An antihyperopic ablation may be carried out around the midperiphery of the cornea if there is significant central ablation.

Complications

- Poor epithelial healing
- Irregular astigmatism
- Corneal haze/scar
- Induced refractive error (most commonly hyperopia, occasionally myopia, astigmatism)
- Recurrence of dystrophy/lesion or herpes simplex keratitis
- Infectious keratitis

Prognosis

- Excellent to fair, depending on the indication for surgery. In general, the more superficial the lesion, the better the results. Lesions can recur; retreatment is often possible.

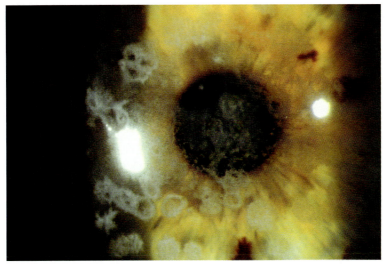

A

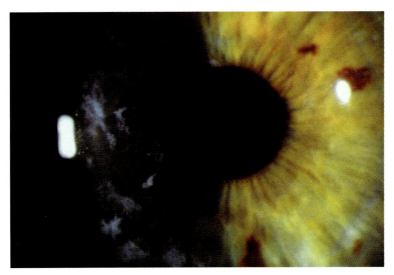

B

Figure 10-6 Excimer laser PTK **A.** *This patient has significant granular dystrophy deposits in the anterior stroma. Fortunately the confluent deposits are rather superficial and amenable to excimer laser treatment.* **B.** *The same eye seen in Figure 10-6A 6 weeks after laser PTK using a 6-mm diameter circular ablation zone. Note the significant clearing of the central opacities. Some of the deeper opacities remain, but do not greatly affect vision.*

CONJUNCTIVAL FLAP

Conjunctival flap surgery is used to resurface a compromised corneal surface. It involves mobilizing the conjunctiva of the eye and securing it down over the cornea. A complete (Gunderson's) or a partial flap can be fashioned.

Indications

- Nonhealing sterile corneal ulcerations (e.g., postinfectious or neurotrophic)
- Chemical injuries with severe ocular surface compromise, if enough healthy conjunctival tissue remains
- Chronic painful bullous keratopathy
- Certain ulcerative keratitis (e.g., Mooren's ulcer, autoimmune corneal melting)

Contraindications

- Corneal perforation
- Active microbial keratitis
- Pain from intractable glaucoma and not from bullous keratopathy

Surgical Technique

- Local anesthesia is used.
- All corneal epithelium and any superficial necrotic tissue are completely removed.
- A superior cornea traction suture is placed.
- Dissection is performed to free a thin layer of superior bulbar conjunctiva from underlying tenons capsule, beginning 12 to 14 mm superior to the limbus.
- A 360-degree peritomy is performed.
- The flap is pulled down toward the inferior limbus and then sutured in place over the cornea superiorly and inferiorly (Figure 10-7A).

Complications

- Flap perforation (buttonhole)
- Insufficient flap to cover cornea
- Flap retraction, often due to excessive traction on the flap (Figure 10-7B)
- Epithelial inclusion cyst

Prognosis

- Very good for stabilization of the corneal surface and comfort. The vision generally does not improve and the cosmetic result is acceptable.

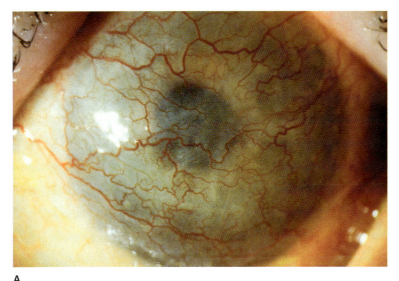

A

B

Figure 10-7   Conjunctival flap   A. *Three months after a Gunderson-type conjunctival flap for herpes zoster neurotrophic keratopathy, the surface is nicely healed and the eye is comfortable with no ongoing inflammation.* **Conjunctival flap complication   B.** *This conjunctival flap developed a buttonhole centrally and subsequent severe flap retraction. Great care must be taken when performing a conjunctival flap to prevent buttonholes and minimize traction on the flap.*

LIMBAL STEM CELL TRANSPLANTATION

Limbal stem cell transplantation is performed to replace limbal stem cells that have been lost or damaged. It may be performed alone or in preparation for subsequent penetrating keratoplasty.

Indications

- Extensive limbal stem cell deficiency (e.g., chemical burns, aniridia, previous ocular surgery)

Special Considerations

- For uniocular disease, conjunctival limbal autograft from the fellow eye can be performed.
- For bilateral ocular disease, the options are a cadaveric or living-related conjunctival limbal allograft. In these cases, systemic immunosuppression is required.

Surgical Technique

- Superficial keratectomy is performed to remove epithelium and existing pannus.
- Circumferential keratectomy of one-third depth, measuring 2 clock hours by 3 mm wide is performed at the 6 and 12 o'clock limbal regions.
- From the donor eye, two pieces of similarly-shaped limbal tissue are excised from the limbus, incorporating some conjunctiva supported on corneoscleral tissues.
- Donor tissues are sutured in place (Figure 10-8).
- A tarsorrhaphy, bandage contact lens, or an amniotic membrane overlay graft may aid in corneal reepithelialization.

Complications

- Poor reepithelialization
- Infectious keratitis
- Rejection of limbal stem cells

Prognosis

- Fair. Long-term systemic immunosuppression is generally required unless tissue is from the fellow eye.

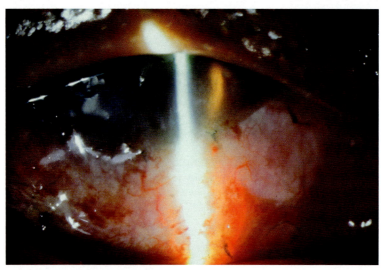

Figure 10-8 Limbal stem cell transplant *Two limbal stem cell grafts have been sutured into the inferior limbus of this eye with severe surface disease. (Photo courtesy of Sadeer Hannush, M.D.)*

AMNIOTIC MEMBRANE TRANSPLANTATION

Amniotic membrane grafts are used to aid in conjunctival and corneal reepithelialization. As amniotic membranes have anti-inflammatory and antifibroblastic properties, and contain healthy extracellular matrix, they can act as a bandage to heal a variety of ocular surface diseases. However, they cannot replace lost or damaged limbal stem cells.

Indications

- Symptomatic bullous keratopathy
- Persistent epithelial defect
- Nonhealing sterile ulcers
- Conjunctival defect or shortage (e.g., Stevens-Johnson syndrome, ocular cicatricial pemphigoid)
- Chemical or thermal burns

Surgical Procedure

- Local anesthesia is given.
- Loose corneal epithelium and any superficial necrotic tissue are completely removed.
- For the purpose of providing a healthy extracellular matrix to aid reepithelialization or for replacing conjunctival tissue, the membrane is sutured with the smooth basement membrane side facing upwards. In this case, epithelium must be completely removed from the underlying bed before securing the membrane so that reepithelialization can take place over the amniotic membrane (Figure 10-9).

- For bandage purposes, the amniotic membrane is sutured onto the ocular surface with the basement membrane side facing down against the cornea. Occasionally a large bandage amniotic membrane graft is sutured over a smaller amniotic membrane graft.
- The eye is then patched for 24 to 48 hours and given frequent antibiotic ointment instillation until reepithelialization has taken place. Alternatively, a bandage soft contact lens can be placed or a tarsorrhaphy can be performed.

Complications

- Poor reepithelialization
- Infectious keratitis

Prognosis

- Fair to good, depending on the underlying ocular condition

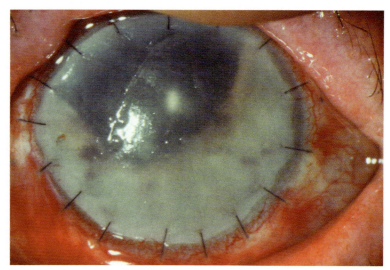

Figure 10-9   Amniotic membrane graft   *A 12-mm diameter circular amniotic membrane graft was performed 1 day prior in this eye with poor visual potential with chronic painful bullous keratopathy. All the corneal epithelium was removed and the membrane was sutured stromal side down with 10-0 nylon sutures. The surface epithelialized over a period of 1 week and the eye has remained comfortable.*

CORNEAL PERFORATION

A corneal perforation is a full-thickness hole in the cornea. If the anterior chamber is flat, the hole should ideally be closed within 24 to 48 hours to prevent significant anterior segment damage.

Etiology

- Infectious stromal keratitis (e.g., bacterial, fungal, herpetic)
- Inflammatory stromal keratitis (e.g., rheumatoid arthritis, other collagen vascular diseases)
- Trauma (e.g., surgically-induced necrotizing sclerokeratitis, burns)
- Neurotrophic keratopathy
- Drugs (e.g., nonsteroidal anti-inflammatory agents, topical corticosteroids)

Symptoms

- Depends on the cause. History is often suggestive of etiology.
- May have acute onset of tearing, redness, decreased vision, pain, photophobia.

Signs

- Preexisting pathology may be seen (e.g., stromal infiltrate, marginal keratolysis).
- Shallow or flat anterior chamber with iris-cornea or lens-cornea contact.
- Positive Siedel's test.
- Disappearance of hypopyon.
- Descemet's folds usually radiating from the site of perforation.
- Iris tissue may occasionally be incarcerated or prolapsing from the perforation and the pupil may become distorted.
- Soft eye, typically, but occasionally the eye can be firm.

Treatment

Pinpoint Perforations (<0.5 mm)
- Eye patch or a soft bandage contact lens.
- If the anterior chamber fails to deepen after 24 hours or if the leakage fails to stop after several days, other measures will have to be considered. Taper and discontinue topical corticosteroids and use aqueous suppressants.

Small and Medium-Sized Perforations (0.5 to 2 mm)
- Cyanoacrylate tissue adhesive (e.g., Histacryl® glue).
- This glue polymerizes in seconds and forms a very firm bond with the tissue. Healing and reepithelialization gradually take place beneath the glue over weeks to months. The glue will then be spontaneously dislodged. Taper and discontinue topical corticosteroids and use aqueous suppressants.

TECHNIQUE
The epithelium and necrotic tissue around the perforation is first removed. The area is dried with a cellulose sponge and a thin layer of glue is applied. A bandage soft contact lens must then be placed for comfort and to prevent the glue from dislodging (Figure 10-10A).

Large Perforations (>2 mm)
- Patch graft for smaller, peripheral perforations. Fresh cornea or cryopreserved cornea or sclera can be used.
- Penetrating keratoplasty for central or larger perforations (Figure 10-10B).

Complications

- Infection, either infectious keratitis or endophthalmitis
- Persistent leak
- Epithelial downgrowth
- Glaucoma, especially if significant peripheral synechiae persist
- Cataract

Prognosis

- Good for small, peripheral leaks which seal spontaneously or with tissue adhesive. Fair to poor for central perforations. Once sealed and healed, central perforations may require a penetrating graft for visual rehabilitation. Prognosis depends greatly on the underlying cause of the perforation.

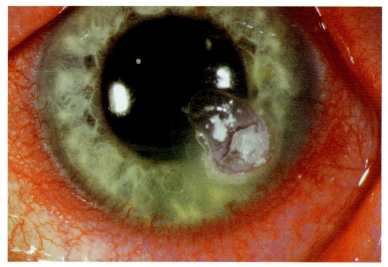

A

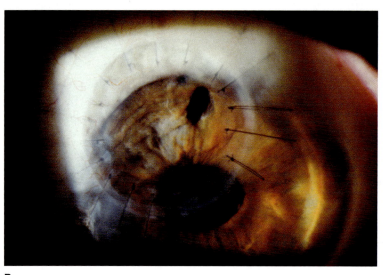

B

Figure 10-10   Cyanoacrylate corneal glue   A. *This eye with a sterile corneal melt and perforation was treated with cyanoacrylate corneal glue to seal the perforation and a bandage soft contact lens. The glue generally remains in place for weeks to months and falls off when the hole has sealed.* **Corneal patch graft   B.** *The eye seen in Figure 9-2E with a sterile corneoscleral melt after cataract surgery associated with the use of postoperative generic diclofenac developed a large perforation and was treated with a patch graft. The graft remains clear and the visual acuity good through a clear visual axis.*

REFRACTIVE SURGERY

Refractive surgery refers to operations that alter the refractive state of the eye to treat refractive errors, commonly myopia, hyperopia, and astigmatism. These operations are usually performed on the cornea and their effects are usually permanent.

Types of Refractive Surgery

Incisional Surgery Radial keratotomy (RK) and astigmatic keratotomy (AK), relaxing and steepening keratotomies.

Laser Surgery Photorefractive keratectomy (PRK) and laser-assisted in-situ keratomileusis (LASIK).

Implant Surgery Intrastromal corneal ring segment (Intacs), intracorneal lens and phakic intraocular lens implantation.

Others Clear lens extraction for high myopia, scleral expansion bands for presbyopia, thermal keratoplasty.

Surgical Principles

RK and AK

- In RK, a variable number of radial incisions of approximately 90% to 95% depth are made using a guarded diamond blade in the paracentral and peripheral cornea. These incisions cause the corneal periphery to bulge outwards which secondarily flattens the central cornea to correct myopia (Figure 10-11A).
- In AK, arcuate or tangential incisions are placed, usually in pairs, perpendicular to the steeper axis of the cornea to produce a flattening effect in that axis.

Relaxing Incisions With or Without Compression Sutures Limbal relaxing incisions can be performed during or after cataract surgery to correct astigmatism. Relaxing incisions can also be performed after corneal transplantation. These incisions are generally performed in the graft–host interface or in the periphery of the graft. These incisions are performed in the steep axis. Compression sutures in the graft–host interface can be used to augment the effect of the relaxing incisions. Limbal relaxing incisions can correct 1 to 3 diopters of astigmatism and relaxing incisions can correct up to 3 to 6 diopters of astigmatism. The addition of compression sutures increases the effect to up to 6 to 10 diopters of astigmatism (Figure 10-11B).

Intacs In Intacs, C-shaped polymethylmethacrylate ring segments are inserted in the corneal periphery for the treatment of low myopia. The intrastromal volume addition causes forward bulging of the anterior surface of the peripheral cornea thereby flattening the central optical zone. The treatment is titratable and potentially reversible. It can correct up to 3 to 4 diopters of myopia, but currently does not correct astigmatism.

PRK In PRK, the corneal epithelium is removed and the central cornea is flattened using an argon-fluoride excimer laser (193 nm). Epithelial-sparing PRK is a variant of PRK in which dilute alcohol is placed on the epithelium to mobilize it. The epithelium is then moved to the side, the surface laser ablation is performed, and then the epithelium is repositioned centrally. It is effective and safe for the correction of myopia of up to 6 to 10 diopters and astigmatism of up to 4 to 5 diopters.

LASIK In LASIK, a partial-thickness, hinged corneal flap is first created using a micro-keratome or femtosecond laser. The flap is folded to one side, excimer laser ablation is carried out on the stromal bed, and then the flap is replaced over the stroma without suturing. It is effective and safe for the correction of myopia of up to 10 to 14 diopters and astigmatism of up to 4 to 5 diopters, depending on the corneal thickness (Figure 10-11C).

Phakic Intraocular Lens (IOL) These are IOLs that are inserted either into the anterior or posterior chamber through a corneal incision for the correction of high myopia or hyperopia. PRK or LASIK may subsequently be performed for residual refractive error (bioptics).

Complications

General
- Undercorrection or overcorrection
- Regression or progression of refractive error
- Infectious keratitis
- Allergy to topical medications
- Glare, halos, decreased quality of vision
- Irregular astigmatism
- Loss of best corrected visual acuity

RK and AK
- RK incisions extending into or across the visual axis: this causes glare, distortion, and induced astigmatism.
- Inaccurate AK incisions: missing the astigmatic axis results in astigmatic undercorrection or induced astigmatism.
- Intraoperative corneal perforation: this can be due to inaccurate pachymetry, the use of an unfamiliar diamond knife, an incorrect depth setting on the knife, altered intraocular pressure, or corneal dehydration during the procedure.
- Epithelial cysts within incision site. Early or late infections can occur in the incisions (Figures 10-11D,E).
- Postoperative rupture at sites of incision after blunt ocular injury.

Relaxing Incisions With or Without Compression Sutures
- Same as RK and AK
- Regression or progression of effect
- Graft rejection
- Dehiscence of graft wound

Intacs
- Corneal perforation: the blade may perforate internally into the anterior chamber or externally through the corneal surface.
- Induced astigmatism: may be due to uneven depth of the intrastromal tunnel or related to the placement of sutures at the site of incision.
- Deposits within the intrastromal tunnel adjacent to the ring segments: the resulting silvery appearance may become obvious even on gross inspection, especially in eyes with dark irides.
- Epithelial cyst formation at the site of incision.

PRK
- Irregular astigmatism: may be due to central island or decentered ablation
- Subepithelial and anterior stromal haze (Figure 10-11F)
- Loss of contrast sensitivity
- Corticosteroid induced glaucoma

LASIK

- Large epithelial defect: may be due to sub-clinical anterior basement membrane dystrophy. This may result in subepithelial haze or scarring and increases the risk of diffuse lamellar keratitis and infection.
- Free or lost cap: free caps may be of normal size or smaller and are typically related to an unusually flat cornea (average keratometry typically <41 diopters) or to lost vacuum suction during the microkeratome pass (Figure 10-11G).
- Irregular or incomplete flaps: these may be related to loss of suction or microkeratome malfunction.
- Buttonholed flap: may be due to an unusually steep cornea (average keratometry typically >48 diopters).
- Penetration into anterior chamber: a result of faulty microkeratome assembly.
- Flap striae: may be microstriae (insignificant) or macrostriae which will need repositioning of flap (Figures 10-11H,I).
- Dislodged flaps: due to trauma or eye rubbing after surgery (Figure 10-11J).
- Irregular astigmatism: due to decentered ablations, central islands, or flap complications.
- Epithelial ingrowth: growth of surface epithelial cells into the flap interface; more common after enhancement procedures (Figure 10-11K).
- Diffuse lamellar keratitis (sands of Sahara syndrome): sterile inflammatory reaction at the level of the flap interface due to a variety of insults, including bacterial endotoxins and meibomian secretions.

- Infection in the interface: often from unusual organisms such as atypical mycobacteria (Figure 10-11L).
- Induced keratectasia: progressive corneal thinning and steepening, generally due to inadequate residual stromal bed thickness after laser ablation. At least 250 mm of residual stromal bed thickness is recommended after lamellar refractive surgery.
- Eyelid trauma and ptosis: from excessively forceful retraction of speculum or from the microkeratome resection.
- Interface haze
- Interface debris
- Dry eyes

Phakic Intraocular Lens

- Induced astigmatism
- Glaucoma
- Pigment dispersion and iritis
- Pupil distortion
- IOL optic incarceration
- Endophthalmitis
- Chronic endothelial damage
- Subsequent difficulty with ophthalmoscopy and cataract surgery
- IOL decentration: this is usually due to an undersized IOL.
- Anterior subcapsular cataract formation: especially with posterior chamber IOL.

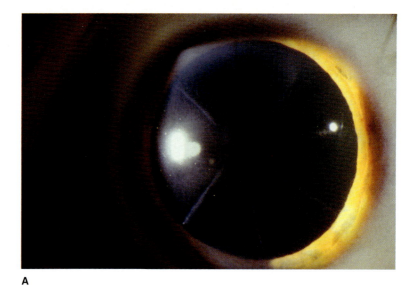

A

B

Figure 10-11   RK   A. *Eight RK incision scars can still be seen 9 years after the procedure for moderate nearsightedness.* **Relaxing incisions and compression sutures   B.** *Relaxing incisions in the graft–host junction were performed from 2 to 5 o'clock and 8 to 11 o'clock. Compression sutures of 10-0 nylon were placed 90 degrees away to augment the effect of the relaxing incisions. Relaxing incisions alone can treat approximately 3 to 6 diopters of astigmatism, while the addition of compression sutures can increase the effect to approximately 6 to 10 diopters. (Continued.)*

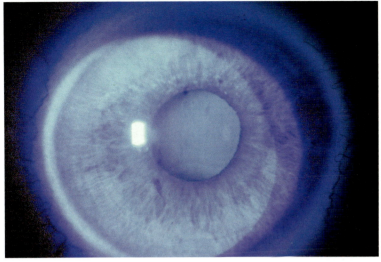

C

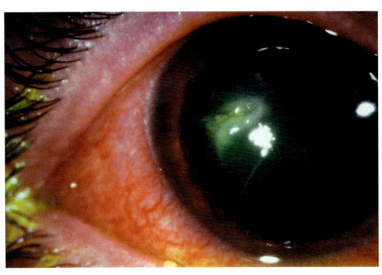

D

Figure 10-11 (cont.) LASIK C. *One day after LASIK for moderate myopia in the right eye, fluorescein dye and the cobalt blue light reveal the edge of the LASIK flap temporally. There is minimal staining.* **RK complication—infectious corneal ulcer D.** *A corneal ulcer is present in the 9 o'clock RK incision. There is surrounding corneal edema and moderate conjunctival injection. It resolved with antibiotic treatment but resulted in corneal scarring and irregularity and decreased vision. (Continued.)*

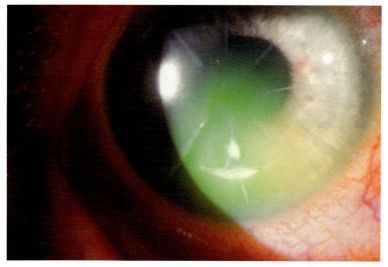

E

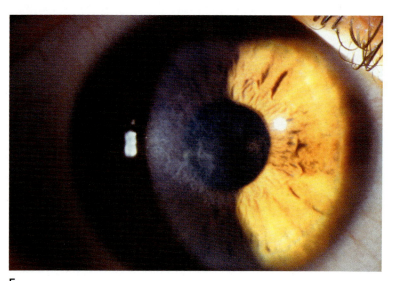

F

Figure 10-11 (cont.)   RK complication—infectious corneal infiltrates   E. *Two dense corneal infiltrates are present in the 6 o'clock radial and astigmatic incisions. Corneal infections in these deep radial/astigmatic keratotomy incisions need to be worked up and treated aggressively to prevent invasion into the anterior chamber and possible endophthalmitis.* **PRK complication— haze   F.** *Moderate haze can be seen several months after PRK for –3 diopters of myopia. It was treated with topical corticosteroids and resolved over the next year. (Continued.)*

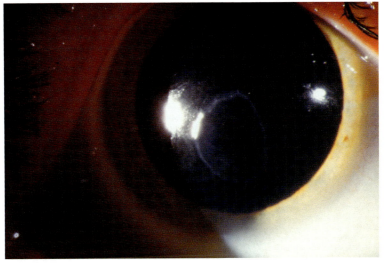

G

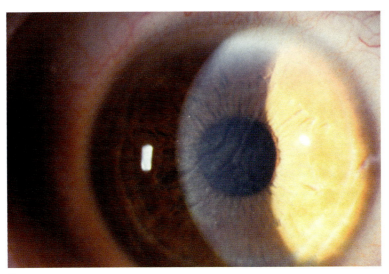

H

Figure 10-11 (cont.)   LASIK complication—small free cap   G. *A small free cap occurred during the microkeratome pass in this eye. The cap was replaced and it healed with scarring, irregular astigmatism, and poor vision.* **LASIK complication—flap striae   H.** *Moderate vertical and oblique striae of the corneal flap are present weeks after LASIK. The flap had been lifted and stretched once without much improvement in the striae. Mild striae (microstriae) do not affect the corneal curvature or the vision significantly while moderate or severe striae distort the curvature and create irregular astigmatism. (Continued.)*

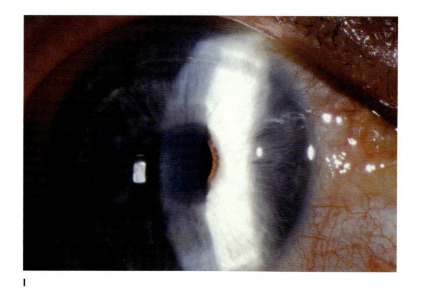

I

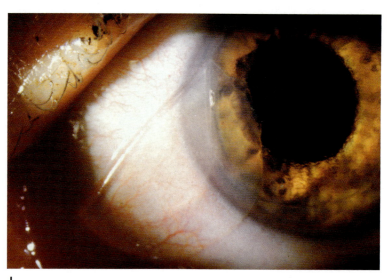

J

Figure 10-11 (cont.) LASIK complication—displaced flap with striae **I.** *This LASIK flap with a nasal hinge is slightly displaced 1 day after surgery. Note the prominent flap gutter superiorly and parallel flap folds from the superior end of the hinge at 3 o'clock. Vision was poor due to irregular astigmatism. It was immediately repositioned and the vision returned to normal, and the flap striae improved but did not completely disappear.* **LASIK complication—dehisced flap** **J.** *This patient was poked in the left eye several months after LASIK, causing a dehiscence of the flap. It is folded on itself but still attached to the cornea at the nasal hinge. It was repositioned immediately, resulting in complete recovery of vision. Care must be taken to remove all epithelium from the corneal stromal side and the underside of the flap before replacing it. (Continued.)*

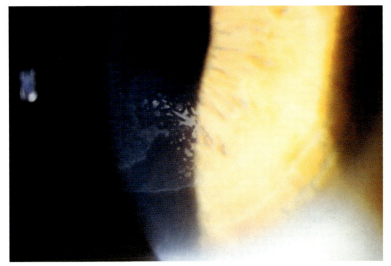

K

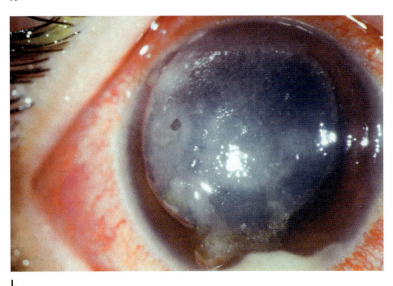

L

Figure 10-11 (cont.) LASIK complication—epithelial ingrowth K. *White epithelial cysts are present under this LASIK flap. This epithelial ingrowth occurs when epithelial cells grow under the flap edge. Risk factors include a displaced flap, epithelial defect, and an enhancement procedure. Ingrowth of 1 to 2 mm not affecting vision can usually be followed. Greater degrees of epithelial ingrowth can cause irregular astigmatism and poor vision or even flap melting and should be removed.* **LASIK complication—interface infectious keratis L.** *A severe atypical mycobacterial infection developed in this eye after LASIK. Small interface spots were noted a few weeks after LASIK. Despite treatment, the infiltrates worsened until they involved almost the entire flap and caused flap melting at the 9 o'clock position. A hypopyon is present inferiorly. The infection was not controlled until the necrotic flap was amputated.*

Chapter 11

TRAUMA

Ocular trauma is a leading cause of blindness in developed countries. Trauma may occur in industrial settings, in sports, or at home. Most of the patients affected are young males and the majority of cases are anterior segment injuries.

CHEMICAL BURN

An ocular chemical burn is an emergency requiring immediate irrigation with water or saline solution at the site of injury for at least 30 minutes. Mechanical removal of foreign particles should also be performed. These actions should be instituted after quickly checking the pH of the tears and repeated at the emergency room even before taking a history or performing an eye examination.

If initial evaluation shows potentially life-threatening respiratory or gastrointestinal involvement, these conditions should be attended to first.

Etiology

- Alkali: examples include sodium hydroxide (lye), calcium hydroxide (lime, cement, plaster), and ammonia.
- Acids: sulfuric acid (battery fluid).
- Mace (chloroacetophenone) and tear gas.
- Organic solvents.
- Detergents.

Symptoms

- Pain, redness, tearing, decreased vision

Signs

Mild to Moderate
- Burns and edema of the eyelid
- Conjunctival injection, chemosis, abrasion
- Punctate or large epithelial defects on cornea (Figure 11-1A)
- Mild anterior chamber activity.

Severe
- Severe burns of the skin of the eyelids.
- Severe chemosis, conjunctival necrosis, conjunctival ischemia (sludging or absence of blood flow through conjunctival vessels) (Figures 11-1B,C,D,E).
- Scleral/limbal ischemia.
- Significant anterior chamber activity.
- Corneal epithelial defects, edema, or melting (Figure 11-1F).
- Poor or no view of the anterior chamber due to corneal haze (Figure 11-1G).
- Intraocular pressure may be low, normal, or elevated in acute stages.
- The degree of limbal ischemia and corneal haziness carries prognostic importance.

Treatment

- Mild cases may be treated on an outpatient basis. Severe injuries may require hospitalization.
- Copious irrigation with normal saline through an intravenous infusion set for at least 30 minutes and repeated every 30 minutes until neutral pH is reached.
- Mechanical removal of foreign particles and debridement of necrotic tissues should be performed with a cotton stick or jeweler's forceps under topical anesthesia.
- Frequent instillation of preservative-free tear drops (q 1 h).
- Cycloplegics (e.g., scopolamine 0.25% or atropine 1% tid).
- Topical antibiotic ointment (e.g., erythromycin, bacitracin, or tetracycline) q 2 h if an eye patch is not used. Pressure patching may aid in re-epithelialization.
- Control intraocular pressure if it is elevated, either with topical drops or oral carbonic anhydrase inhibitors.
- For injuries with significant inflammation and without risk of corneal melting, topical corticosteroid (e.g., dexamethasone 0.1% or prednisolone 1%) q 1 to 2 h may be used during the first week, tapered during the second week, and increased after epithelial healing if necessary.
- Topical acetylcysteine 10% drops qid may help control collagenase activity and corneal melting.
- High-dose vitamin C 1 g po tid and topical ascorbate 10% drops q 1 to 6 h may be helpful in severe alkali burns.
- Doxycycline 100 mg po bid can be used to decrease collagenase activity.
- If there is symblepharon formation, daily sweeping of the fornices with a cotton stick or glass rod should be performed under topical anesthesia to break the adhesions. Alternatively, a scleral shell may be used.
- For progressive corneal melting or perforation, tissue adhesive, amniotic membrane graft, limbal stem cell graft, lamellar patch graft, or penetrating keratoplasty may be necessary.

Complications

- Corneal scarring
- Dry eyes
- Symblepharon
- Cicatricial entropion or ectropion
- Trichiasis or distichiasis
- Punctal stenosis or occlusion
- Limbal stem cell deficiency
- Pannus formation
- Cataract
- Glaucoma

Prognosis

- Dismal to excellent depending on the severity of the injury (Figure 11-1H). In general, alkaline substances cause the most severe injuries because they penetrate tissues easily.

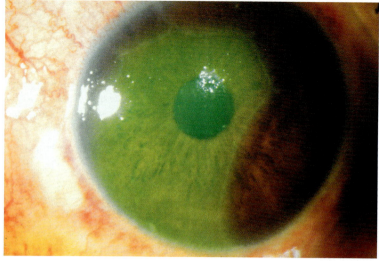

A

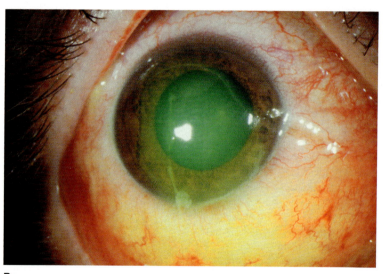

B

Figure 11-1 Chemical burn   ***A.*** *A mild acid injury caused a large corneal abrasion, which has been stained with yellow fluorescein dye. There is minimal to no conjunctival blanching and the cornea is essentially clear. Mild chemical burns generally resolve without serious consequences.* ***B.*** *A sulfuric acid injury occurred to this patient's right eye. There is a large central and inferior corneal epithelial defect and mild inferior conjunctival blanching. (Continued.)*

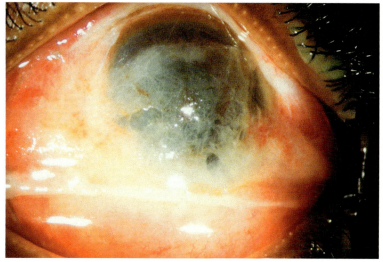

C

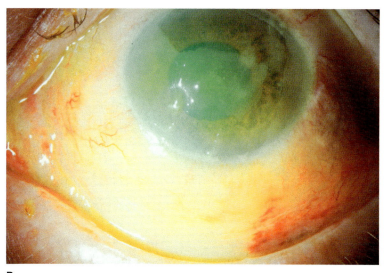

D

Figure 11-1 (cont.)   Chemical burn   C. *This eye withstood a battery acid (sulfuric acid) injury. There is moderate conjunctival blanching and mucus adherent to the conjunctiva and cornea.*
D. *The left eye of the patient seen in Figure 11-1B has a much more extensive sulfuric acid injury. The epithelium is necrotic and has already sloughed off of the superior cornea. There is extensive conjunctival and scleral blanching inferiorly and nasally. (Continued.)*

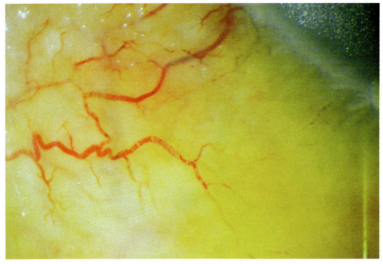

E

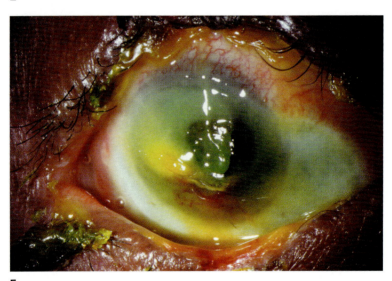

F

Figure 11-1 (cont.)   Chemical burn   E. *High magnification view of the same eye as seen in Figure 11-1D demonstrates ischemia of the conjunctiva and sclera. There is segmentation of the red blood cells indicating lack of blood flow. The greater the degree of ischemia, the worse the prognosis.* **F.** *A severe lye (sodium hydroxide) injury caused extensive ischemic damage in the lower two thirds of the eye. The cornea has undergone necrosis centrally leading to a perforation requiring an emergent corneal transplant. This alkali injury eventually resulted in enucleation. (Continued.)*

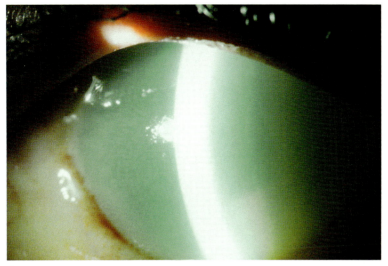

G

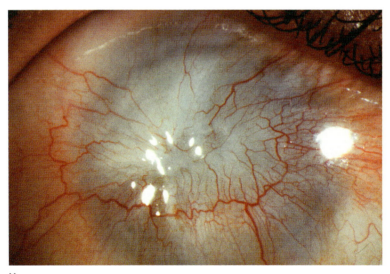

H

Figure 11-1 (cont.)   Chemical burn   G. *Twelve days after a severe alkali injury, the conjunctiva and sclera remain blanched and the cornea is opaque. There has been no reepithelialization of the damaged cornea or conjunctiva.* **H.** *Many years after a severe chemical burn, the cornea remains totally scarred and vascularized.*

THERMAL AND ELECTRICAL BURNS

THERMAL BURNS

Thermal burns can be mild to severe and can occur at any age. Cigarette burns are not uncommon in small children whose eyes are at hand level of a person holding a cigarette.

Etiology

- Curling irons
- Cigarettes, especially children
- Flames
- Hot liquids
- Molten metals

Symptoms

- Pain, redness, decreased vision

Signs

- Thermal burns on skin of eyelids
- Conjunctival injection, chemosis, epithelial defects
- Punctate or large epithelial defects on cornea
- A white area of cauterized epithelium (Figure 11-2A)

In Severe Cases
- Anterior chamber reaction
- Corneal haze and edema
- Limbal or scleral ischemia, corneal or scleral perforation (Figure 11-2B)

Treatment

- Removal of foreign bodies and debridement of devitalized tissues.

- Topical antibiotic ointment to prevent infection and to lubricate the ocular surface (e.g., erythromycin, bacitracin, ciprofloxacin q 2 to 6 h).
- Cycloplegics (e.g., cyclopentolate 1% or scopolamine 0.25% tid).
- Pressure patching, lateral tarsorrhaphy, or amniotic membrane graft should be considered for large or nonhealing epithelial defects.
- Topical corticosteroids to reduce inflammation and prevent symblepharon formation during the first 1 to 2 weeks, bearing in mind they can potentiate corneal melting.

Complications

- Corneal scarring
- Irregular astigmatism
- Decreased vision
- Infectious keratitis

Prognosis

- Depends on the severity of the injury, especially the exact cause of the burn and duration of contact. Short-contact burns, such as those from curling irons and cigarettes, have an excellent prognosis. Molten metal that adheres to the cornea causes a much more substantial injury. Eyelid damage can cause exposure problems and long-term difficulties with corneal healing.

ELECTRICAL BURNS

Ocular electrical burns usually result from electrical injuries to the head or a lightning strike. In addition to corneal and scleral burns, they can also cause acute uveitis. The lens is frequently involved and cataracts may develop many months to years later. Eyelid damage can cause exposure problems and long-term difficulties with corneal healing.

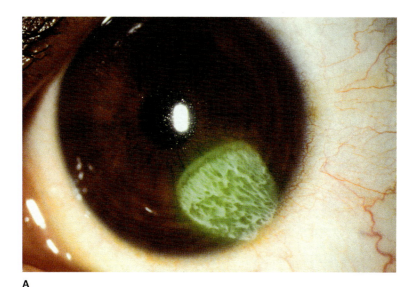

A

B

Figure 11-2   Thermal injury   A. *A curling iron briefly touched this cornea causing coagulation of the corneal epithelium and turning it white. It can be removed mechanically or it will slough off naturally. Generally, these eyes recover without sequelae as the amount of time the heat is in contact with the cornea is minimal.* **Electrical injury   B.** *An electrical injury caused a localized area of scleral melt with uveal prolapse. Additionally, the electrical injury produced necrosis of a large portion of upper eyelid tissue resulting in severe exposure. The eye was treated with a scleral patch graft and eyelid skin grafting.*

ULTRAVIOLET KERATOPATHY (ARC WELDER'S FLASH)

Severe, painful punctate keratopathy can result hours after exposure to significant ultraviolet light exposure.

Etiology

• Usually caused by welding or using a sunlamp without proper use of protective eyewear.

Symptoms

• Symptoms usually develop 6 to 10 hours after the exposure.
• Pain, photophobia, foreign body sensation, tearing, redness, and decreased vision.

Signs

• Spasm of eyelids in severe cases
• Punctate epithelial erosions, especially in the interpalpebral regions (Figure 11-3)
• Eyelid edema, conjunctival hyperemia

Treatment

• Preservative-free artificial tears q 2 to 3 h.
• Topical antibiotic drops qid and antibiotic ointment at bedtime. For more severe cases, topical antibiotic ointment qid will provide more lubrication and comfort.
• Cycloplegics (e.g., cyclopentolate 1% or scopolamine 0.25% tid).
• Pressure patching for severe epithelial erosions.
• Emphasize to the patient the importance of protective eyewear.

Complications

• Rarely, infectious keratitis

Prognosis

• Typically excellent

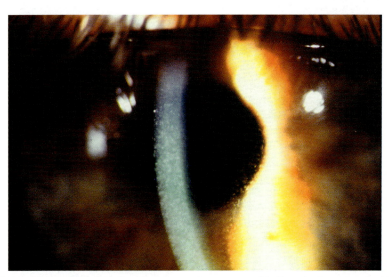

Figure 11-3   Welder's flash   *Significant central punctate epitheliopathy is present in this patient 6 hours after welding without adequate eye protection. (Courtesy of Irving Raber, M.D.)*

CORNEAL ABRASION

Corneal abrasions result from corneal surface trauma that causes removal of a portion of the epithelial layer.

Etiology

- Mechanical trauma (e.g., fingernail, paper edge, tree branch)
- Chemical injuries, medicamentosa keratitis
- Foreign body
- Contact lens
- Misdirected eyelashes
- Neurotrophic or exposure keratopathy
- Iatrogenic (e.g., after removal of corneal sutures, epithelial debridement)

Symptoms

- Pain, especially on blinking; foreign body sensation; photophobia; tearing; redness; often decreased vision.
- Topical anesthetic drops relieve the pain (and facilitate the eye examination).

Signs

- Epithelial defect that may be detected grossly or under the slit-lamp. It is easily seen with fluorescein dye using the cobalt blue light (Figures 11-4A,B).

Treatment

- Search for and remove any foreign body in the conjunctival fornices and under the upper eyelid.
- Epilate any misdirected eyelashes
- Topical antibiotic ointment (e.g., erythromycin, tetracycline, bacitracin, or ciprofloxacin) q 2 to 6 h. Topical antibiotic drops may be used if abrasion is small or if patient finds that ointments blur vision.
- Cycloplegics (e.g., cyclopentolate 1% or scopolamine 0.25% tid).
- Pressure patching for large defects. Small defects generally do not require patching.
- For traumatic or contact lens–induced abrasions, bandage contact lenses and patching are contraindicated because they increase the risk of infection. A topical antibiotic with good gram-negative coverage (e.g., ciprofloxacin, tobramycin, polymyxin B/neomycin/gramicidin) should be used.

Complications

- Corneal scar
- Infectious keratitis
- Decreased vision
- Recurrent erosions

Prognosis

- Generally excellent. Patients need to be followed closely until the abrasion heals, especially those at higher risk of infection, such as after contact lens–related and vegetable matter–related trauma.

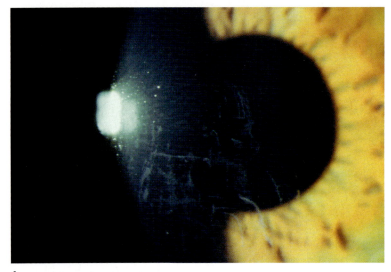

A

B

Figure 11-4   Corneal abrasion   A. *A tennis ball hit the eye of this 12-year-old boy causing multiple linear corneal abrasions. It also caused a traumatic iritis.* **B.** *A triangular corneal abrasion is evident superiorly with the cobalt blue light after fluorescein stain. There is some punctate epithelial staining surrounding the abrasion.*

CORNEAL AND CONJUNCTIVAL FOREIGN BODIES

Ocular trauma can result in foreign bodies that remain embedded in the cornea or conjunctiva.

Types

- Bits of metal or rust
- Glass fragments
- Plastic fragments
- Dirt
- Insect hairs
- Vegetative matter (high risk of microbial contamination)

History and Symptoms

- It is important to determine from the history whether the foreign body was propelled at high speed into the eye (e.g., metal on metal hammering), which may suggest an intraocular foreign body. The type of foreign body may also be obtained from the history.
- Foreign body sensation, tearing, redness, decreased vision.
- Topical anesthetic drops can relieve the pain and facilitate examination of the eye.

Signs

- Foreign bodies may be seen on the cornea or conjunctiva. They may be superficial, subconjunctival, or embedded in the corneal stroma or sclera (Figures 11-5A,B,C).
- Rust ring or sterile infiltrate may surround a corneal foreign body (Figure 11-5D).
- Anterior chamber reaction may be present, but is usually mild.
- Fluorescein staining may reveal linear corneal abrasions, typically seen with foreign bodies retained on the superior tarsal conjunctiva.
- Eyelid eversion or double eversion with a Desmarres' retractor may reveal foreign bodies trapped in the conjunctival fornices.
- In the presence of conjunctival/scleral/corneal laceration, significant anterior chamber activity, iris tears, or lens opacities, it is imperative to exclude an intraocular foreign body, ideally by CT scan.

Treatment

- An accurate assessment of the depth of penetration is important prior to removing a deep corneal foreign body. If it has partially penetrated into the anterior chamber, it should be removed in the operating room under adequate anesthesia.
- For nonperforating foreign bodies, they can be removed under topical anesthesia with a cotton-tipped applicator, a foreign body spud, or a pair of jeweler's forceps.
- The residual rust ring may be removed with a burr. Deeper rust rings can be removed later, after they have spontaneously migrated to the surface (Figure 11-5E).
- The resultant epithelial defect is treated with topical antibiotic ointments bid (e.g., tetracycline, bacitracin, ciprofloxacin) or drops qid (e.g., trimethoprim/polymyxin, ciprofloxacin, levofloxacin, ofloxacin).
- Certain deep, nonexposed, inert foreign bodies may not need removal if they are located away from the visual axis (e.g., glass fragments).
- Subconjunctival foreign bodies may require a conjunctival incision to facilitate removal. A scleral laceration may be difficult to rule out if significant subconjunctival hemorrhage is present. In this case, surgical exploration may be necessary.
- Topical corticosteroids may be used after reepithelialization and in the absence of infection to reduce scarring if the visual axis is involved.
- After removal of vegetative foreign bodies, patients have to be followed closely for signs of infection, especially fungal keratitis.

Complications

- Corneal scarring
- Infectious keratitis
- Recurrent erosions

Prognosis

- Depends on the severity of the injury. Conjunctival and superficial, noncentral corneal foreign bodies generally cause few problems. Deep, central foreign bodies can cause scarring and impaired vision.

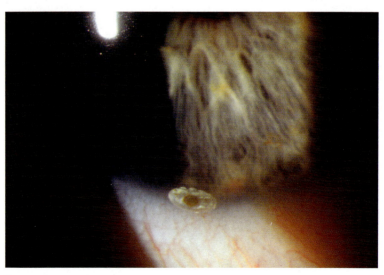

A

Figure 11-5 Corneal foreign body A. *A small portion of seed cover is adherent to the inferior limbal area, causing a foreign body sensation. It was easily removed at the slit-lamp with jeweler's forceps. (Continued.)*

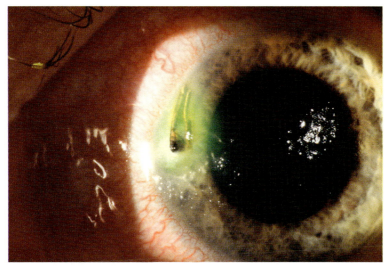

B

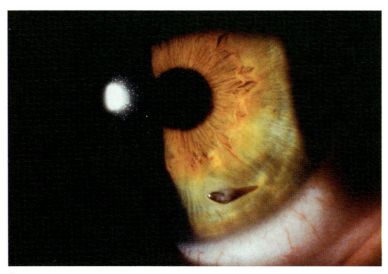

C

Figure 11-5 (cont.) **Corneal foreign body** **B.** *A large fragment of a nail had broken off while it was being hammered, and the fragment was deeply lodged in the corneal periphery. A prime concern was whether it had perforated full-thickness cornea. Gentle gonioscopy revealed intact stroma behind the nail. It was removed at the slit-lamp in the minor surgery suite so that suturing of the wound could be done if necessary. There was no leak of aqueous humor and minimal wound gape, so it was left unsutured and healed well.* **C.** *A deeply-embedded thorn was present in the corneal periphery. Gentle gonioscopy revealed no full-thickness corneal break. Caution must be used when removing friable foreign bodies to extract the entire object. (Continued.)*

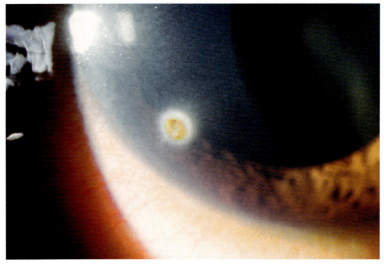

D

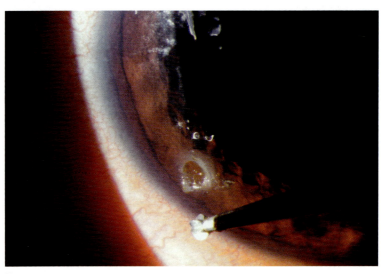

E

Figure 11-5 (cont.)   Corneal rust ring   D. *A small, brown rust ring with underlying corneal infiltrate remains after a metallic foreign body was removed with a foreign body spud. Small, localized infiltrates associated with foreign bodies are typically sterile, but need to be followed closely for infection.* **E.** *The rust ring and most of the infiltrate seen in* **Figure 11-5D** *were carefully removed with a small, hand-held, battery-operated rust ring drill. Care needs to be taken to remove most if not all of the rust while not going too deep into the corneal stroma. A small amount of rust deep in the stroma should be left in place rather than risk corneal perforation.*

SUBCONJUNCTIVAL HEMORRHAGE

Hemorrhage from a conjunctival blood vessel into the subconjunctival space can cause mild to severe bright red discoloration of the conjunctiva.

Etiology

- Traumatic hemorrhage may be associated with hyphema and chemosis. May occur after ocular surgery.
- Hypertension.
- Associated with bleeding disorders and the use of anticoagulants, when it may also be associated with periocular cutaneous ecchymosis.
- Spontaneous hemorrhage is by far the most common type. The hemorrhage is usually unilateral, but when precipitated by coughing or straining, it may be bilateral.

Symptoms

- Usually asymptomatic and noticed by patient incidentally
- Red eye, mild discomfort

Signs

- Sectorial hemorrhage under the conjunctiva (Figure 11-6).

Differential Diagnosis

- Kaposi's sarcoma: a reddish-purple, slightly elevated, vascular lesion beneath the conjunctiva. Suspect in patients with AIDS.
- Conjunctival or scleral laceration/globe rupture: suspect in the presence of more severe injury.

Treatment

- Complete eye examination of both eyes if there is a history of ocular trauma.
- Reassurance, artificial tears for lubrication. Patient should be told it may look worse over the days after hemorrhage as it expands before it resolves over days to weeks.
- Refer to the family doctor for systemic evaluation if recurrent.

Complications

- None

Prognosis

- Excellent

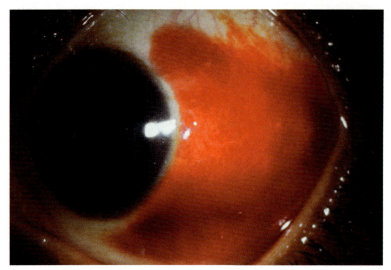

Figure 11-6 Subconjunctival hemorrhage *Blunt trauma to the eye caused a large localized subconjunctival hemorrhage temporally in this left eye. It often spreads over the first few days after the hemorrhage and appears to have become more serious to the patient.*

CORNEOSCLERAL LACERATION AND WOUND DEHISCENCE

Trauma can cause lacerations of the cornea and/or sclera in addition to rupture of a previous ocular surgery wound.

Etiology

- Industrial accidents (e.g., projectile metallic/nonmetallic foreign bodies, glass fragments, nails, sharp instruments)
- Road traffic accident (e.g., injury by windshield)
- Home accidents (e.g., sharp edges on toys)
- Assault (e.g., knives)
- Traumatic wound rupture (most commonly after cataract surgery, penetrating keratoplasty, and trabeculectomy)

History and Symptoms

- It is important to determine from the history whether the foreign body was propelled at high speed into the eye (e.g., metal on metal hammering), which may suggest intraocular foreign bodies. History of ocular surgery.
- Pain, redness, decreased vision.

Signs

- Examination of the eye should be done cautiously without exerting pressure on the globe so as to prevent herniating intraocular contents through the wound. Detailed examination is often deferred until the time of surgical repair.
- The eye is usually extremely soft (hypotony).
- Blurred vision: visual acuity should be documented for medicolegal reasons.
- Subconjunctival hemorrhage, chemosis, corneal edema.
- Prolapse of uveal tissues through the wound.
- Shallow or flat anterior chamber with or without hyphema.
- Pupil distortion, iridodialysis, cyclodialysis.
- Ruptured anterior lens capsule, subluxed lens, cataract, vitreous presentation may be seen.

Diagnosis

- The diagnosis is usually apparent on gross or slit-lamp examination (Figures 11-7A–K).
- Siedel's test may be used to confirm that a laceration is partial-thickness. In full-thickness lacerations, it can also help to assess the rate of aqueous leakage and wound stability.
- Occasionally, full-thickness scleral lacerations may be masked by the overlying subconjunctival hemorrhage and chemosis. These may require surgical exploration to determine the extent of injury.
- Computed tomography, x-ray, and/or B scan to look for intraocular foreign bodies and retinal detachment as needed.

Treatment

- Once the initial evaluation is completed, the eye should be protected with an eye shield.
- No ointment should be applied to the eye.
- Tetanus prophylaxis should be given and intravenous antibiotics started immediately.
- Analgesics and antiemetics should be given to minimize pain and vomiting.
- Small lacerations may be observed, treated with a pressure patch or bandage contact lens, or sealed with tissue adhesives. A persistent leak or decrease in anterior chamber depth requires surgical repair.
- Surgical repair for larger lacerations should be carried out as soon as possible under general anesthesia, usually depending on when the patient ate last.
- If the attempt at repairing the laceration fails due to a severely traumatized eye, enucleation may be considered, but is generally performed as a secondary procedure to allow time for further assessment and patient counseling. In eyes with severe damage and poor visual

potential, enucleation should be considered within 2 weeks to reduce the chance of sympathetic ophthalmia.

Treatment of Late Complications

Corneal Scars

INDUCED IRREGULAR ASTIGMATISM Fitting with rigid gas-permeable contact lenses after all corneal sutures are removed.

DENSE OPACITIES Rotational autograft, lamellar or penetrating keratoplasty.

Diplopia and Glare from Pseudopolycoria or Corectopia Contact lens with peripheral tinting.

Unsightly Corneal Opacities in Eyes Without Visual Potential Prosthetic contact lenses or cosmetic penetrating keratoplasty.

Complications

- Infectious keratitis
- Endophthalmitis
- Corneal scarring
- Cataract
- Iris and damage and pupillary irregularity
- Retinal detachment
- Decreased vision or blindness
- Epithelial downgrowth

Prognosis

- Dismal to good, depending directly on the severity of the injury and postoperative complications.

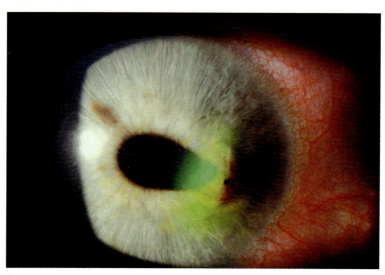

A

Figure 11-7 Corneal laceration A. *While being hammered, a nail hit this eye and caused a full-thickness corneal laceration. Note the distorted pupil and iris incarceration in the corneal wound. This injury required repair in the operating room, which included repositing the iris and closing the laceration with 3 sutures. The patient was treated with systemic antibiotics to prevent infection. (Continued.)*

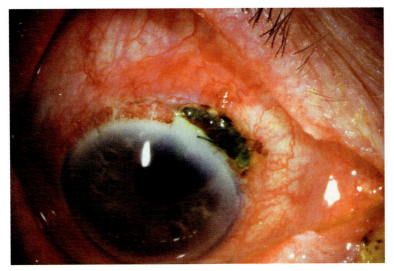

B

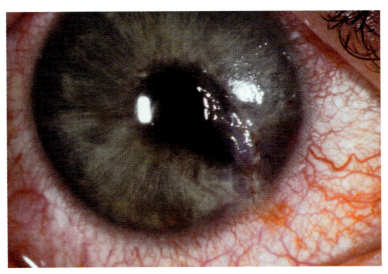

C

Figure 11-7 (cont.) Cataract surgery wound dehiscence **B.** *Many years after an extracapsular cataract extraction, this eye withstood blunt trauma that caused a partial dehiscence of the cataract wound. Iris prolapse can be seen from the 1 o'clock to 2:30 o'clock positions. The blue haptic of the posterior chamber intraocular lens can also be seen exiting from the wound. The lens and iris were repositioned and the wound closed emergently in the operating room.* **Corneal laceration** **C.** *A full-thickness corneal laceration with pupil distortion and iris prolapse is evident. It was repaired emergently. (Continued.)*

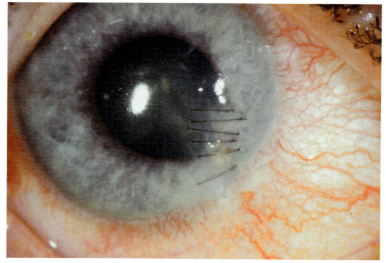

D

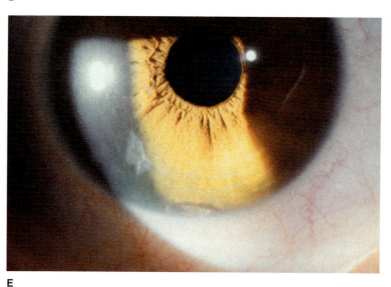

E

Figure 11-7 (cont.) Corneal laceration **D.** *Ten days after surgical repair of the eye seen in Figure 11-7C. The iris was reposited in the eye and the laceration required 6 10-0 nylon sutures to close.* **Corneal laceration and intraocular foreign body** **E.** *After an automobile accident, a small, healed corneal laceration is evident in the midperiphery at 7 o'clock. A glass foreign body can be seen in the inferior angle. While glass is typically inert and generally does not cause significant inflammation, it was removed surgically through an inferior limbal approach to prevent corneal and other intraocular damage. (Continued.)*

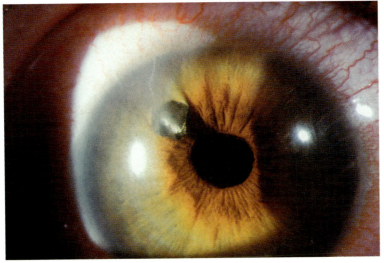

F

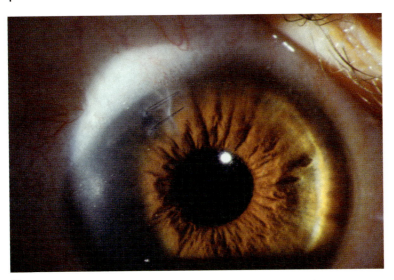

G

Figure 11-7 (cont.)   Corneal laceration and intraocular foreign body   F. *A large fragment of metal is resting on the iris after a hammering injury. The corneal laceration is seen just superior to the foreign body. Interestingly, the patient had undergone a LASIK procedure 6 months prior. The laceration was repaired with two interrupted sutures, being very careful not the disturb the LASIK flap edge. A limbal incision was made superiorly to remove the metal shard.* **G.** *Five months after surgical repair of the eye seen in Figure 11-7F. The vision returned to preinjury levels and the LASIK flap was unaffected. (Continued.)*

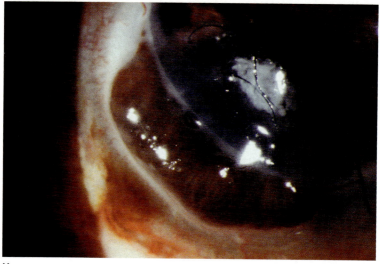

H

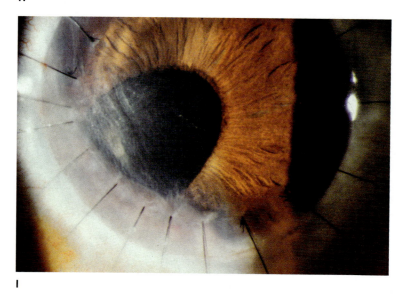

I

Figure 11-7 (cont.)   Corneal transplant wound dehiscence   H. *Several months after undergoing a corneal transplant, the patient fell and hit his eye, causing a wound dehiscence. Five broken sutures and significant iris prolapse can be seen. It was emergently repaired by repositing the iris and resuturing the wound.* **I.** *Five days after wound repair in the eye seen in Figure 11-7H, the wound is secure. While no iris tissue was amputated, the iris sphincter was damaged so the pupil was still distorted. The graft is remarkably clear. (Continued.)*

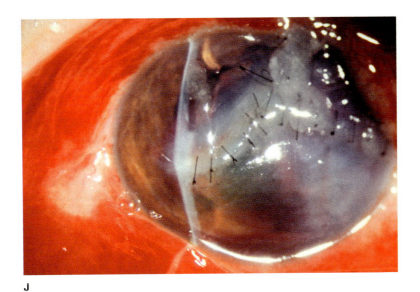

J

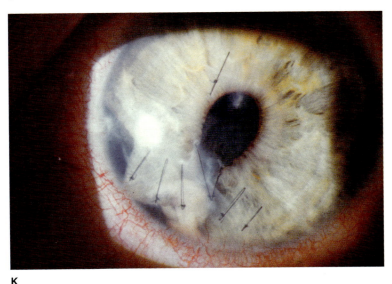

K

Figure 11-7 (cont.)   Corneal laceration   J. *This severe corneal laceration with iris and lens damage was caused by a heron peck to the eye. It was repaired with multiple interrupted sutures. Mucus is seen on the corneal surface and blood is present in the anterior chamber.* **K.** *This corneal laceration was repaired 4 months previously. Note the partial-thickness laceration superior to the pupil required 1 suture as it was gaped, while the inferior full-thickness laceration required 8 sutures to close. There were also two separate iridodialyses from 7 to 9 o'clock.*

TRAUMATIC HYPHEMA

Trauma causes bleeding into the anterior chamber, which is termed a hyphema.

Etiology

- Trauma damages the iris, typically at the iris root, causing bleeding.

Symptoms

- Redness, pain, photophobia, decreased vision
- Often a history of blunt trauma

Signs

Microhyphema   Red blood cells suspended in the anterior chamber

Hyphema   Red blood cells layered or a clot in the anterior chamber angle (Figures 11-8A,B)

- May be associated with more extensive ocular damage

Treatment

- Consider hospitalization.
- Check for sickle trait or disease.
- Bed rest or limited activity and an eye shield.
- Atropine 1% tid.
- Consider topical corticosteroids (e.g., prednisolone 1% q 2 to 6 h).
- Consider aminocaproic acid (50 mg/kg q 4 h, maximum 30 g/day) orally for 3–5 days.
- Treat elevated intraocular pressure (IOP), especially in patients with sickle trait or disease.
- Avoid aspirin, nonsteroidal anti-inflammatory agents and other medications that may increase bleeding.
- Consider evacuation of hyphema if persistent or IOP remains elevated.

Complications

- Glaucoma
- Cataract
- Iris damage
- Corneal blood staining

Prognosis

- Fair to excellent, depending on the extent of associated ocular injury. Elevated IOP can cause severe damage in sickle cell trait or disease patients. Need to monitor for late development of glaucoma.

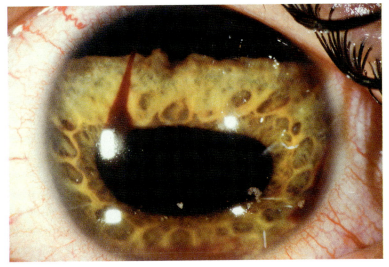

A

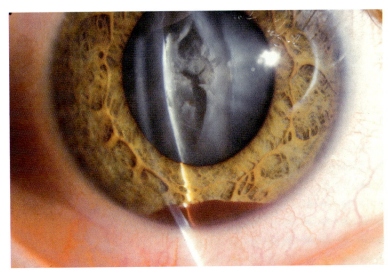

B

Figure 11-8   Hyphema   A. *Blunt trauma to the eye caused an iridodialysis superiorly. Previous bleeding had caused blood to layer inferiorly (hyphema). A stream of active bleeding is coming from the superior angle. Remarkably, there was no cataract and the vision was quite good.* **B.** *Blunt trauma caused bleeding in the anterior chamber, leading to layering of blood in the inferior angle. It also caused a break in the anterior lens capsule and a secondary cataract.*

EPITHELIAL DOWNGROWTH

Epithelial downgrowth occurs when ocular surface epithelium grows into the eye through a full-thickness wound.

Etiology

- Penetrating injuries
- Ocular surgery (e.g., penetrating keratoplasty, cataract surgery, trabeculectomy)

Symptoms

- Pain, photophobia, tearing, redness, often decreased vision

Signs

- The epithelium forms a membrane that covers the corneal endothelium, anterior chamber angle, iris, ciliary body, lens, and capsular bag. Often a wavy line on the corneal endothelial surface can be seen. When on the iris, the membrane causes flattening of the normal iris crypts (Figure 11-9A).
- Corneal decompensation and severe, intractable glaucoma may result.
- Argon laser photocoagulation produces white burns rather than charring of epithelial membranes on the iris surface and helps make the diagnosis and delineate the extent of the membrane (Figure 11-9B).
- Occasionally, a fluid-filled cyst with a clear anterior wall, similar to a primary iris stromal cyst, may form in the anterior chamber.

Treatment

- Extensive surgery is needed to effect removal via excision, laser ablation, or cryotherapy of the intraocular membrane and involved tissues.
- Repair of wound fistula.
- Glaucoma drainage implant for treatment of glaucoma.

Complications

- Corneal decompensation
- Intractable glaucoma

Prognosis

- Even with extensive surgery, the prognosis is poor.

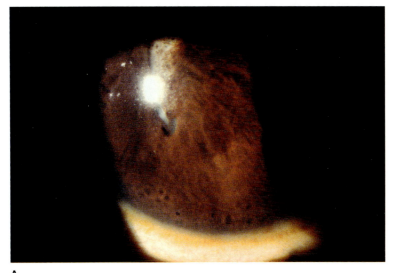

A

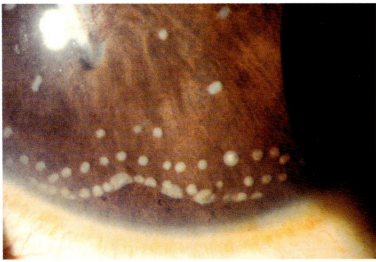

B

Figure 11-9   Epithelial downgrowth   A. *Two years after surgical repair of a ruptured globe near the superior limbus, the patient returns with a membrane that has grown across the pupil and has covered 95% of the iris. The membrane has flattened the iris crypts. The edge of the epithelial downgrowth membrane can be seen inferiorly as can a small degree of normal peripheral iris.*
B. *An argon laser was used to delineate the extent of the epithelial downgrowth in the eye seen in Figure 11-9A. The argon laser creates distinct white spots in the membrane but not in normal iris. The edge of the membrane is seen inferiorly.*

DESCEMET'S DETACHMENT

Small tears in Descemet's membrane that do not progress or cause visual symptoms are commonly seen after ocular surgery. Tears in Descemet's membrane can lead to a Descemet's detachment and subsequent corneal edema and poor vision.

Etiology

- Ocular surgery, most commonly cataract surgery
- Rarely, trauma

Symptoms

- Discomfort, decreased vision

Signs

- A tear in Descemet's membrane, typically originating at the surgical wound
- Undulating or scrolled Descemet's membrane in the anterior chamber separated from the posterior stroma (Figure 11-10A)
- Corneal edema

Treatment

Small Detachments These can be followed and may resolve spontaneously over weeks to months.

Larger Detachments or Those Not Resolving Spontaneously
- If Descemet's membrane is not scrolled, a bubble of air or long-acting gas (e.g., 18% to 20% sulfur hexafluoride) can be injected into the anterior chamber to push the membrane against the posterior stroma (Figure 11-10B). Proper head posture is required postoperatively to reattach the membrane. The condition may resolve within days or take weeks.
- If Descemet's membrane is scrolled, it must first be unscrolled surgically. An air bubble or long-acting gas can then be injected into the anterior chamber or it may be repaired with suturing, but suturing can further tear the membrane.

Complications

- Corneal scarring
- Corneal edema

Prognosis

- Many unscrolled Descemet's detachments will resolve spontaneously. Long-acting intraocular gas has a good success rate, especially in unscrolled detachments. Scrolled detachments are more difficult to repair. Chronic edema may require a penetrating keratoplasty to achieve good vision.

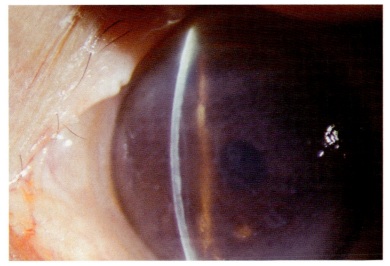

A

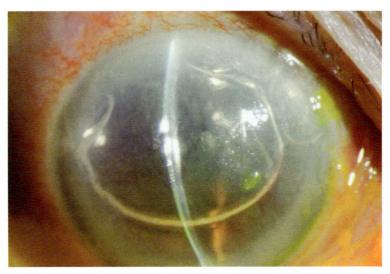

B

Figure 11-10   Descemet's detachment   A. *Slit-lamp beam view demonstrates an arc of detached Descemet's membrane behind the edematous cornea. The patient developed this Descemet's detachment at the time of temporal clear corneal cataract surgery 1 month prior.* **B.** *A nonexpansile concentration of sulfur hexafluoride gas was injected into the anterior chamber to tamponade Descemet's membrane against the back of the cornea to reattach it in the eye seen in Figure 11-10A. Within days, Descemet's membrane was reattached and the corneal edema had resolved.*

INDEX

Page numbers followed by *f* and *t* indicate figures and tables, respectively.

C

Calcium concretions, 43, 44*f*
Calcium deposits, in band keratopathy, 129, 130*f*, 131*f*
Candida keratitis, 153, 154*f*
Capillary hemangioma, 59
Carcinomas, 53, 56*f*
Carotid-cavernous sinus fistulas, 59–60, 61*f*
Cat scratch disease, and Parinaud's oculoglandular syndrome, 22, 23*f*
Cataract(s), Wilson's disease and, 208
Cataract extraction, 248, 249*f*–251*f*
 wound dehiscence and, 301*f*
Chalazion, 4, 5*f*, 49
Chalchosis, 208
Chandler's syndrome, in iridocorneal-endothelial syndrome, 145
CHED. *See* Congenital hereditary endothelial dystrophy
Chemical burn, 282–283, 284*f*–287*f*
Chemicals, and ophthalmia neonatorum, 24
Chlamydia trachomatis
 and conjunctivitis, 12
 and ophthalmia neonatorum, 24, 25*f*
Chlamydial conjunctivitis, 12, 13*f*
Choroiditis, and herpes zoster keratitis, 172
Chrysiasis, and corneal crystals, 137
Churg-Strauss syndrome, 49
Cicatricial pemphigoid, ocular, 219–220, 220*f*, 221*f*
Ciprofloxacin, and corneal deposits, 137, 138*f*
Climatic droplet keratopathy, 133
Coats' white ring, 133, 135*f*
Cogan-Reese syndrome, in iridocorneal-endothelial syndrome, 145
Cogan's microcystic dystrophy, 93, 94*f*–95*f*
Cogan's syndrome, and interstitial keratitis, 175, 176
Collagen vascular diseases, 215, 216*f*
 and necrotizing scleritis, 238
Coloboma, iris, 80, 81*f*
Colobomatous microphthalmos, 66, 67*t*
Concretions, calcium, 43, 44*f*
Congenital anterior keratectasia, 69, 69*f*
Congenital anterior staphyloma, 69, 69*f*
Congenital hereditary endothelial dystrophy (CHED), 122, 123*f*
Conjunctival amyloidosis, 43, 44*f*
Conjunctival calcium concretions, 43, 44*f*

Conjunctival cyst, 58, 58*f*
Conjunctival degenerations, 40–61
Conjunctival epithelial melanosis, 45, 46*f*
Conjunctival flap, 266, 267*f*
Conjunctival foreign bodies, 293–294, 294*f*–296*f*
Conjunctival infections and inflammations, 2–39
Conjunctival intraepithelial neoplasia, 53, 54*f*–55*f*
Conjunctival lesions
 benign amelanocytic, 49–52
 melanocytic, 45–48, 46*f*, 47*f*, 48*f*, 49*f*
 potentially malignant amelanocytic, 53–57
Conjunctival mass lesions, 40–61
Conjunctival papilloma, 40
Conjunctivitis. *See also* Keratoconjunctivitis
 adult inclusion, 12, 13*f*
 allergic, 26, 27*f*, 37*f*, 201
 bacterial
  gonococcal, 8, 9*f*
  nongonococcal, 6, 7*f*
 chlamydial, 12, 13*f*
 follicular, 16, 17*f*
 giant papillary, 30, 201, 205*f*
 and herpes zoster keratitis, 171
 ligneous, 18, 19*f*
 limbal vernal, 31*f*
 neonatal, 24, 25*f*
 toxic, 36, 37*f*, 201
 viral, 10, 11*f*
Contact lens-associated superior limbic kerato-conjunctivitis, 202, 206*f*
Contact lens complications, 201–204, 205*f*–207*f*
Contact lens keratopathy, 202, 206*f*
Contact lens overwear syndrome, 202
Cornea
 abrasion of, 291, 292*f*
 biopsy of, 262, 262*f*
 ectatic conditions of, 82–92
 foreign bodies in, 293–294, 295*f*–296*f*
 infections and inflammations of, 148–207
 iron deposits in, 139, 140*f*, 141*f*
 shape anomalies of, 62–72
 size anomalies of, 62–72
 transplantation of, 252–253, 254*f*–259*f*
  rejection of, 231, 232*f*–234*f*
  wound dehiscence and, 304*f*
Cornea farinata, 125, 127*f*

Epithelial downgrowth, 231, 308, 309*f*
Epithelial iron deposits, 139, 140*f*
Epithelial keratitis
  herpes simplex, 161, 162*f*–163*f*
  in viral conjunctivitis, 10, 11*f*
Erosions
  punctate epithelial, 179, 180*f*
  recurrent corneal, 192, 193*f,* 194*f*
Erythema multiforme major, 222, 223*f*–224*f*
Excimer laser phototherapeutic keratectomy
  (PTK), 264, 265*f*
Exposure keratopathy, 188, 189*f*
External hordeolum, 4
Extrascapular method, of cataract extraction,
  248
Eyelid eversion
  with chalazion, 4, 5*f*
  with floppy eyelid syndrome, 34, 35*f*

F

Fabry's disease
  and cornea verticillata, 136
  and vascular lesions, 59
Factitious keratoconjunctivitis, 36, 37*f*
Ferry's line, in corneal iron deposits, 139
Filamentary keratopathy, 186, 187*f*
Fistulas
  carotid-cavernous sinus, 59–60, 61*f*
  dural-sinus, 59–60
Fleischer's ring, 84*f*
  in corneal iron deposits, 139
Floppy eyelid syndrome, 34, 35*f*
Follicular conjunctivitis, 16, 17*f*
Foreign bodies
  corneal and conjunctival, 293–294, 294*f*–296*f*
  corneal laceration and, 302*f,* 303*f*
Fuchs' dystrophy, 116–117, 117*f*–118*f*
Fuchs' marginal keratitis, 40
Fungal keratitis, 153, 154*f*–155*f*
Fusarium keratitis, 153

G

Gammopathies, monoclonal, and corneal
  crystals, 137
Geographic herpes simplex ulcer, 170
Ghost dendrites, 161, 163*f*
Giant papillary conjunctivitis (GPC)
  with contact lens use, 201, 205*f*

Gillespie's syndrome, 78
Glaucoma
  congenital, 122
  infantile, 68
Gonococcal bacterial conjunctivitis, 8, 9*f*
GPC. *See* Giant papillary conjunctivitis
Graft rejection, 231, 232*f*–234*f*
Granular dystrophy, 101, 102*f*–104*f*
Granuloma(s), 49, 50*f*
  pyogenic, 4, 49, 50*f*
Granulomatous diseases, and necrotizing
  scleritis, 238

H

Haab's striae, 68, 68*f*
Haemophilus influenzae, and bacterial conjunc-
  tivitis, 6
Hay fever conjunctivitis. *See* Allergic conjunc-
  tivitis
HBID. *See* Hereditary benign intraepithelial
  dyskeratosis
Hemangioma, capillary, 59
Hematologic disorders, 59
Hemorrhage, subconjunctival, 297, 298*f*
Hemorrhagic lymphangiectasia, 59
Hereditary benign intraepithelial dyskeratosis
  (HBID), 49, 52*f*
Herpes, primary ocular, 159, 160*f*
Herpes simplex epithelial keratitis, 161,
  162*f*–163*f*
Herpes simplex keratitis, 159–170
  reactivation of, 231
Herpes simplex virus type 2, and ophthalmia
  neonatorum, 24
Herpes zoster ophthalmicus, 171
Herpes zoster virus (HZV) keratitis, 171–172,
  172*f*–174*f*
Hordeolum
  external, 4
  internal, 4, 5*f*
HSV. *See* Herpes simplex virus keratitis
Hudson Stahli's line, in corneal iron deposits,
  139
Hydrops, in keratoconus, 82, 87*f*
Hypercholesterolemia, and corneal crystals,
  137
Hyperlipidemia, and corneal crystals, 137
Hyperplasia, reactive lymphoid, 53, 57*f*
Hypersensitivity, staphylococcal, 229, 230*f*

Hyphema
  and corneal blood staining, 139, 141*f*
  traumatic, 306, 307*f*
HZV. *See* Herpes zoster virus keratitis

I

Iatrogenic cysts, 58
ICE syndrome. *See* Iridocorneal-endothelial
    syndrome
Immunologic conditions, 208–234
Infantile glaucoma, 68
Infections
  conjunctival, 2–39
  corneal, 148–207
Infectious crystalline keratopathy, 137, 138*f*
Inflammations
  conjunctival, 2–39
  corneal, 148–207
Intacs, 273, 274
Internal hordeolum, 4, 5*f*
Interstitial keratitis, 175–176, 176*f*–177*f*
Intraepithelial neoplasia, 40
Intraocular lens (IOL)
  implantation of, 248, 249*f*–251*f*
  phakic, 273–274, 275
Involutional changes, 124–128
IOL. *See* Intraocular lens
Iridocorneal-endothelial (ICE) syndrome, 145,
    146*f*–147*f*
Iris, 235–247
  atrophy of, in iridocorneal-endothelial syn-
      drome, 145, 146*f*, 147*f*
  cysts of, 243, 244*f*
  tumors of, 245, 246*f*–247*f*
Iris coloboma, 80, 81*f*
Iris nevus, 245, 246*f*
  in iridocorneal-endothelial syndrome, 145
Iris pigment epithelial cysts, 243, 244*f*
Iris stromal cysts, 243, 244*f*
Iron deposits
  corneal, 139, 140*f*, 141*f*
  epithelial, 139, 140*f*

K

Kaposi's sarcoma, 59
Kayser-Fleischer ring, 142, 142*f*, 208, 209*f*
Keratectasia, congenital anterior, 69, 69*f*

Keratectomy
  excimer laser phototherapeutic, 264, 265*f*
  superficial, 263, 263*f*
Keratitis
  Acanthamoeba, 156, 157*f*–158*f*
  Aspergillus, 153
  bacterial, 148–149, 150*f*–152*f*
  Candida, 153, 154*f*
  disciform, 164, 165*f*–167*f*
  epithelial
    herpes simplex, 161, 162*f*–163*f*
    in viral conjunctivitis, 10, 11*f*
  Fuchs' marginal, 40
  fungal, 153, 154*f*–155*f*
  Fusarium, 153
  herpes simplex, 159–170, 231
  herpes zoster virus, 161, 171–172, 172*f*–174*f*
  interstitial, 175–176, 176*f*–177*f*
  medicamentosa, 36, 37*f*
  metaherpetic, 170, 170*f*
  microbial, 148, 204
  microsporidial, 198
  necrotizing stromal, 168, 169*f*
  neurotrophic, 170, 170*f*
  non-necrotizing stromal, 164, 165*f*–167*f*
  nonsyphilitic interstitial, 175–176
  peripheral ulcerative, 225
  pseudomonal, 148, 151*f*
  sterile, 204, 207*f*
  streptococcal, 148
  syphilitic interstitial, 175–176
  ulcerative, peripheral, 225
Keratoconjunctivitis. *See also* Conjunctivitis
  atopic, 28, 29*f*
  contact lens-associated superior limbic, 202,
      206*f*
  factitious, 36, 37*f*
  superior limbic, 32, 33*f*, 201–202, 206*f*
  toxic, 36, 37*f*
  vernal, 28, 30, 31*f*
Keratoconjunctivitis sicca, 183, 184*f*–185*f*
Keratoconus, 82–83, 83*f*–87*f*
  localized posterior, 73, 77*f*
Keratoglobus, 91, 92*f*
Keratopathy
  actinic, 133
  band, 129, 130*f*–131*f*
  bullous, 116, 195, 196*f*, 197*f*
  climatic droplet, 133
  contact lens, 202, 206*f*